D1063064

COMMUNICATION SKILLS FOR NURSES

Student Survival Skills Series

Survive your nursing course with these essential guides for all student nurses:

Calculation Skills for Nurses
Claire Boyd
9781118448892

Medicine Management Skills for Nurses
Claire Boyd
9781118448854

Clinical Skills for Nurses
Claire Boyd
9781118448779

Care Skills for Nurses
Claire Boyd
9781118657386

Communication Skills for Nurses
Claire Boyd and Janet Dare
9781118767528

Study Skills for Nurses
Claire Boyd
9781118767528

[redacted]

COMMUNICATION SKILLS
FOR NURSES

Claire Boyd
RGN, Cert Ed
Practice Development Trainer

Janet Dare
Practice Development Teacher, Assessor, IQA
North Bristol NHS Trust

WILEY Blackwell

This edition first published 2014
© 2014 by John Wiley & Sons, Ltd

Registered office:
John Wiley & Sons, Ltd, The Atrium, Southern Gate, Chichester, West Sussex, PO19 8SQ, UK

Editorial offices:
9600 Garsington Road, Oxford, OX4 2DQ, UK
The Atrium, Southern Gate, Chichester, West Sussex, PO19 8SQ, UK
111 River Street, Hoboken, NJ 07030-5774, USA

For details of our global editorial offices, for customer services and for information about how to apply for permission to reuse the copyright material in this book please see our website at www.wiley.com/wiley-blackwell

The right of the author to be identified as the author of this work has been asserted in accordance with the UK Copyright, Designs and Patents Act 1988.

All rights reserved. No part of this publication may be reproduced, stored in a retrieval system, or transmitted, in any form or by any means, electronic, mechanical, photocopying, recording or otherwise, except as permitted by the UK Copyright, Designs and Patents Act 1988, without the prior permission of the publisher.

Designations used by companies to distinguish their products are often claimed as trademarks. All brand names and product names used in this book are trade names, service marks, trademarks or registered trademarks of their respective owners. The publisher is not associated with any product or vendor mentioned in this book. It is sold on the understanding that the publisher is not engaged in rendering professional services. If professional advice or other expert assistance is required, the services of a competent professional should be sought.

The contents of this work are intended to further general scientific research, understanding, and discussion only and are not intended and should not be relied upon as recommending or promoting a specific method, diagnosis, or treatment by health science practitioners for any particular patient. The publisher and the author make no representations or warranties with respect to the accuracy or completeness of the contents of this work and specifically disclaim all warranties, including without limitation any implied warranties of fitness for a particular purpose. In view of ongoing research, equipment modifications, changes in governmental regulations, and the constant flow of information relating to the use of medicines, equipment, and devices, the reader is urged to review and evaluate the information provided in the package insert or instructions for each medicine, equipment, or device for, among other things, any changes in the instructions or indication of usage and for added warnings and precautions. Readers should consult with a specialist where appropriate. The fact that an organization or Website is referred to in this work as a citation and/or a potential source of further information does not mean that the author or the publisher endorses the information the organization or Website may provide or recommendations it may make. Further, readers should be aware that Internet Websites listed in this work may have changed or disappeared between when this work was written and when it is read. No warranty may be created or extended by any promotional statements for this work. Neither the publisher nor the author shall be liable for any damages arising herefrom.

Library of Congress Cataloging-in-Publication Data
Boyd, Claire, author
Communication skills for nurses / Claire Boyd, Janet Dare.
1 online resource.
Includes bibliographical references and index.
Description based on print version record and CIP data provided by publisher; resource not viewed.
ISBN 978-1-118-76750-4 (ePub) – ISBN 978-1-118-76751-1 (Adobe PDF) – ISBN 978-1-118-76752-8 (pbk.)
I. Dare, Janet, author. II. Title.
[DNLM: 1. Nurse-Patient Relations. 2. Communication. 3. Nursing Assessment. WY 88]
RT23
610.7301′4–dc23

2014023322

A catalogue record for this book is available from the British Library.

Wiley also publishes its books in a variety of electronic formats. Some content that appears in print may not be available in electronic books.

Cover image courtesy of Visual Philosophy
Chapter opener image: © iStockphoto.com/Squaredpixels
Cover design by Visual Philosophy

Set in 9/12pt Trade Gothic LT Std by Aptara Inc., New Delhi, India
Printed and bound in Malaysia by Vivar Printing Sdn Bhd

1 2014

Contents

Preface

This book is designed to assist the student healthcare worker in the skill of communication, a fundamental component of effective nursing care. It is designed to give a quick, snappy overview of communication theories, skills and techniques. The book incorporates many exercises to check understanding, and is done in a simple-to-follow step-by-step approach. Chapters end with quizzes to relate everything learned to practice. The aim of this book is to start the individual on their journey of nursing study right up to graduation. It has been compiled by quotes and tips from student nurses themselves: a book by students for students.

Claire Boyd
Bristol
April 2014

Introduction

Communication can take many forms, such as verbal or written. It is quite simply the transfer of information among or between people. However, it is not that simple, as communication, especially in the nursing profession, can be a complicated process. In nursing practice we often have a great deal of information to give or send to others, and we need to do this effectively. Successful communication has three major components:

1. A sender
2. A receiver
3. A message

Whenever we communicate, we should always be aware that there are factors which could influence how our message may be interpreted. Variables will need to be considered, such as the following.

1. Who we are communicating with, be they children, adult patients, colleagues or patients with learning disabilities.
2. The setting in which the communication occurs, such as in hospital, the maternity ward or in a service user's own home.
3. The sender's and/or receiver's past experiences.
4. The sender's and/or receiver's personal perceptions (if known).
5. The timing of the message.

In health care, breakdown in communication may result in devastating results. For example, important information may not be conveyed, such as treatment plans or medications. Let's look at the scenario. You are looking after a patient in a day case unit who has just undergone a minor surgical procedure. After handover and looking at this patient's observations, which have been plotted on an observations chart, everything looks fine, although the person is a little tachycardiac (their heart rate is fast). Then the poor patient vomits. It had not been communicated to you that the patient told the previous nurse that they felt nauseous and had asked for an anti-emetic. This is an example of a breakdown in communication, which caused a negative outcome. Quite frankly, this should not have occurred.

It should never be forgotten that we, the carer, are in a very privileged position caring for our charges – a patient, or in the maternity setting, in the mental health sector or with children or babies – wherever we work.

I remember from my student nurse training being told that communication is 80% non-verbal. We need to observe individuals, paying attention to body language, eye contact, tone of voice and facial expressions. For example, many of you will be performing pain management observations and you will no doubt come across individuals who tell you that their pain is 'OK' when their body language screams that they are in severe pain. Of course, it is a patient's right to refuse analgesia but often these patients will tell you later that they did not want to disturb the nurses, seeing how busy everybody was, and they did not want to be a nuisance.

Much has been written of late, and with good reason, about the lack of care and compassion in nursing. We need to put the human faith back into the profession. Show the patient that we do care, that we are listening.

It is every patient's right to complain, and they should, as we need to know where we are going wrong. Don't lose heart as there are *many* wonderful examples of nurses and midwives doing a sterling job, often in difficult circumstances. And they often go well beyond the normal course of duty. Always strive to be the best that you can and remember why you came into this caring profession.

Janet Dare and I have put together this communications book, giving you, the carer, a quick, easy-to-read book to help you during your training as a student nurse (and beyond), assistant practitioner or healthcare assistant, covering many aspects of the skill of communication. Student nurses have helped us with this book: telling us what they wanted to be included.

We have looked at nursing aspects of communication from the different sectors of nursing, covering those caring for adults, children and maternity. Throughout the chapters we have incorporated actvities to reinforce your learning. At the end of each chapter you will also have Test your Knowledge questions with the answers at the back of the book.

Remember, patients may not always remember our names, but they will remember how they were treated, and that should be with kindness, care and compassion.

Good caring!

Acknowledgements

As always, first acknowledgements go to the student nurses who have helped to make this book possible. As with the other books within the Student Survival Skills series, it is their tips and quotes that have been used throughout the book.

Thanks also go to Janet Dare (Practice Development Teacher/Assessor/IQA) for her assistance with putting this book together.

Thank you to Jane Hadfield (Head of Learning and Development) and to all my friends and colleagues in Staff Development Department at North Bristol NHS Trust. Thanks also to Magenta Styles (Executive Editor at Wiley Blackwell) for first approaching me in this exciting project and to all my friends at Wiley Blackwell, including Nik Prowse (freelance copy-editor) for copy-editing the manuscript and to Mirjana Misina (Project Manager), Madeleine Hurd (Associate Commissioning Editor), Catriona Cooper (Project Editor) and James Schultz (Project Editor). Also a big 'thank you' to Simon Boyd for indexing all the books in the Student Survival series for me.

Thanks also go to the Parliamentary and Health Service Ombudsman for permission to use information from the document *Listening and Learning – the Ombudsman's Review of Complaint Handling by the NHS in England 2009–10*, and also to the National Blood Transfusion Committee for permission to use the front cover of the booklet *Amazing You – Let's Learn About Blood with Billy Blood Drop.*

Lastly, thanks to my family for all their assistance, especially Rob for the photographs and graphs, Simon for the indexing and to David and Louise.

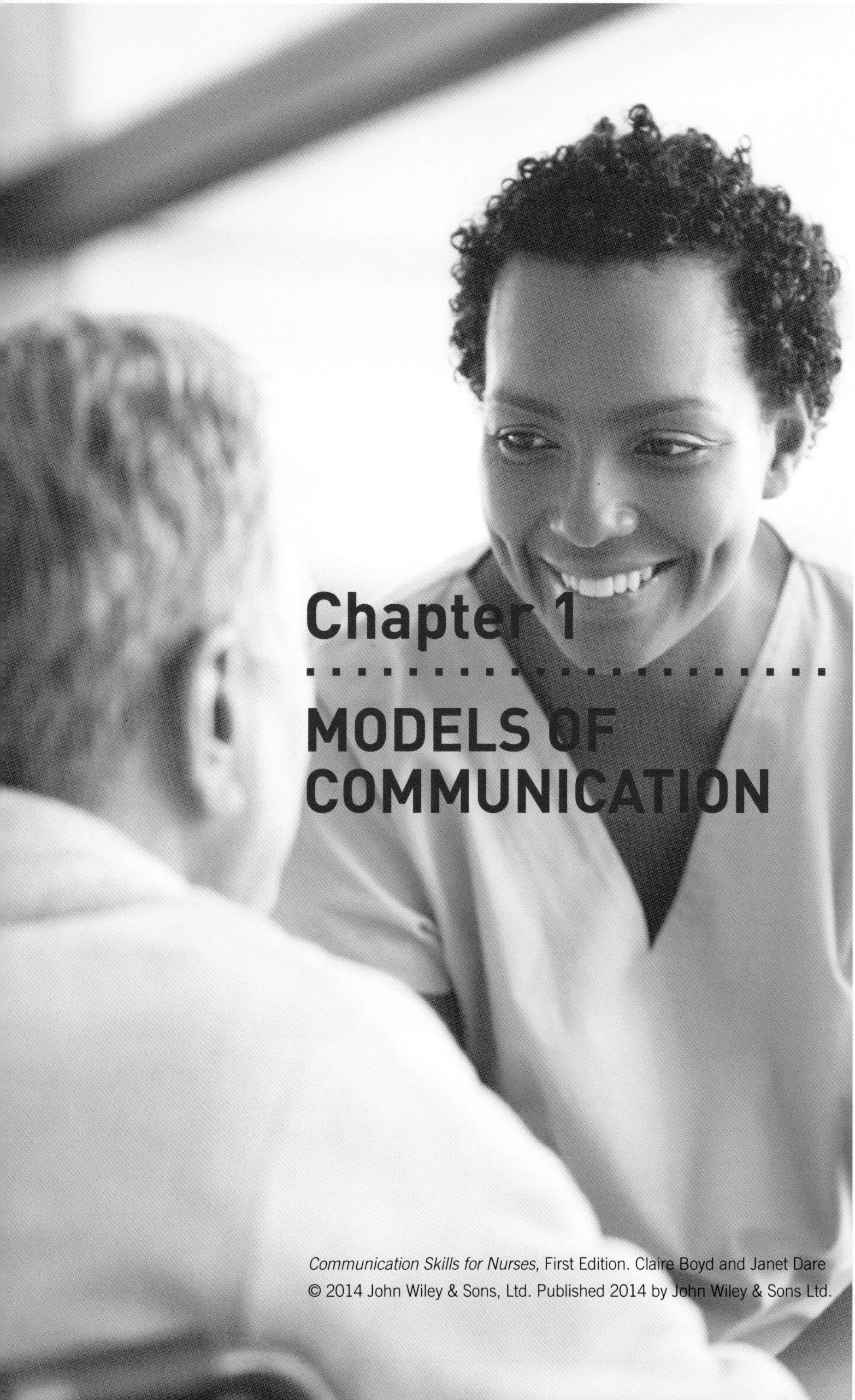

Chapter 1

MODELS OF COMMUNICATION

Communication Skills for Nurses, First Edition. Claire Boyd and Janet Dare
© 2014 John Wiley & Sons, Ltd. Published 2014 by John Wiley & Sons Ltd.

LEARNING OUTCOMES

This chapter will explore communication models that are used frequently as part of a nurse's role.

WHAT IS A COMMUNICATION MODEL?

A communication model is chiefly a process in which information is channelled, then imparted by the sender to the receiver through a medium. When the receiver gets the information they decode the message and may give the sender feedback.

Theorists have analysed the communication process many times and how individuals interact with each other. There are different models of communication that are relevant to a nurse. These are the **linear**, **interactive** and **transactional** models.

Linear Model

The best-known model of communication is the one devised by Shannon and Weaver (1949) and was originally known as 'a mathematical model of communication'. It is a simple linear model that is easily understood.

GLOSSARY

Linear
Arranged in or extending along a straight or nearly straight line or in one direction.

Linear communication consists of a sender creating a message. They send it to the receiver without any feedback. See Figure 1.1.

This model has five main parts:

- information source: where the message is produced,
- transmitter: where the message is encoded (relayed),

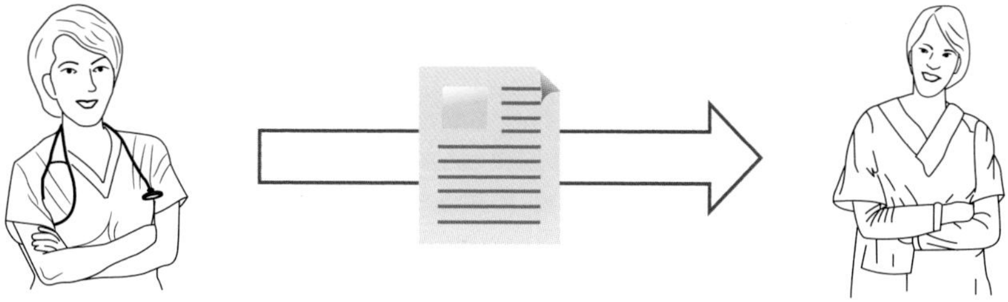

Figure 1.1 A linear model of communication. Adapted from: Shannon and Weaver (1949).

- channel: the carrier of the signal,
- receiver: where the message is decoded,
- destination: where the message ends up.

What this model is suggesting is that during a conversation between two people, at any one time only one person is expressing and sending the information, and the second person is only receiving and absorbing the information. When the information is received and decoded the roles may be reversed, and the second person becomes the sender and the first person the receiver. An example of linear communication is a letter or an email.

One of the advantages of Shannon and Weaver's model is that it is simple and easily understood, and can be applied to most types of communication. However, this type of model has been challenged because it does not take into account simultaneous interaction and transactional feedback. An example of this could be when we try to communicate with people from different cultures; in such cases, the message is relayed by one or more of our five senses (sight, touch, hearing, taste or smell). We observe the listener's body language and if they have not heard our message or it has been misinterpreted then we are able to adapt our communication or adjust our tone of voice to accommodate the listener.

Communication relies on the active participation of both sender and receiver, and cannot be accurately represented by a linear system.

Interactive Model

Wilbur Schramm was one of the early theorists to demonstrate a circular model of communication. He proposed that both the sender and receiver interpret the message, rather than assessing the message's meaning (see Figure 1.2).

Schramm (1955; cited in Wood 2009) saw communication as a two-way process with both the speaker and the listener providing and receiving verbal or non-verbal feedback. Both the speaker and the listener take turns to speak and listen to each other. Other characteristics of messages that impact communication between two individuals are intonation and pitch patterns, accents, facial expressions, quality of voice and gestures. This model also indicates that the speaker and listener communicate better if they have had the same experiences. However, this may mean that both the receiver and sender are limited by their experience.

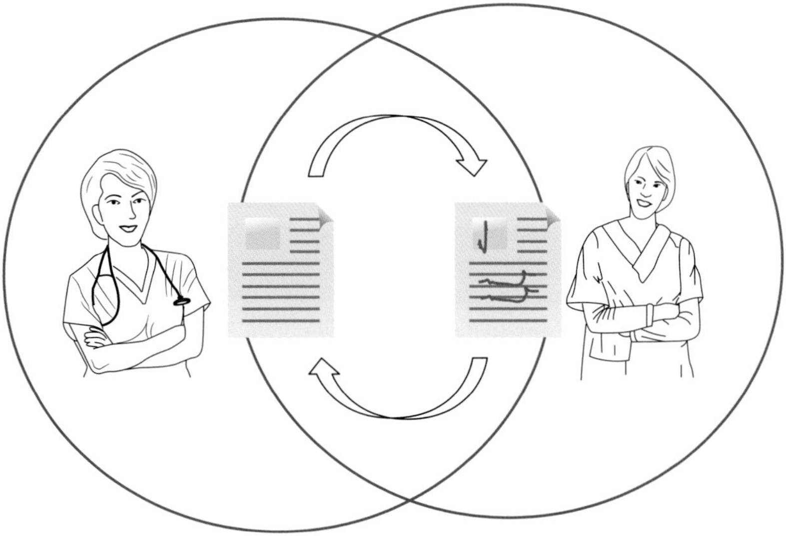

Figure 1.2 An interactive model of communication. Adapted from: Schramm (1954).

Nevertheless, there must be some experience common to both in order for the communication to be useful and for the intended message to be conveyed. For example, if you were asking someone who did not speak the same language as you if they wanted sugar in their coffee, you would most probably point to the sugar and then the cup of coffee, hoping that the other individual has had some common experience of putting sugar in their coffee. However, if the receiver comes from a culture where sugar is not used, then your communication will be ineffective.

Two people from completely different cultures who speak different languages and who have no common experiences may find that communication becomes nearly impossible without help from a third party such as a translator or an interpreter.

Common ground or mutual understanding is important in communication and essential for interpersonal communication.

Transactional Model

The transactional model builds on the interactive model by adding non-verbal communication methods such as gestures, eye contact, use of silence, positioning, facial expressions and body language. It demonstrates that communication is an ongoing and continuously changing process. You are changing, the people with whom you are communicating are changing and your environment is also continually changing as well. Each person in the communication process reacts depending on factors such as their background, prior experiences, attitudes, cultural beliefs and self-esteem.

Figure 1.3 shows a transactional model of communication that takes into account 'noise' or interference in communication as well as the time factor.

As you can see from the diagram, the outer lines of the model indicate that communication happens within a shared **field of experience**. This could be that you have

Figure 1.3 A transactional model of communication. Adapted from: Wood (2009).

worked in the same department or that you know the same person.

The transactional model displays communication interactions as ongoing negotiations of meaning. As already mentioned, non-verbal expressions take on additional importance when you are communicating with people from completely different cultures, speaking different languages and with no common experiences with which to take part in this negotiation of meaning.

Individuals come to a communication interaction with their own field of experience. This includes things like personal culture, history, gender, social influences and experience. Your field of experience is the frame of reference that you bring to each situation that you encounter. At times, individuals' fields of experiences overlap and they share things in common.

Other times, individuals' fields of experiences do not overlap; and because they share no common past experiences, it is difficult to negotiate meaning.

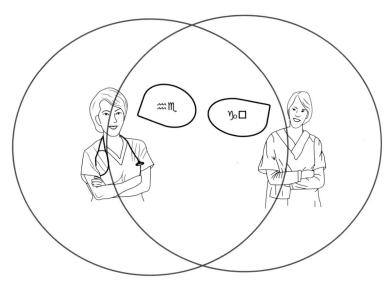

TEST YOUR KNOWLEDGE

1. What is a communication model?
2. What type of model was identified by Shannon and Weaver (1949)?
3. The transactional model builds on the interactive model by adding what into the communication?

KEY POINTS

- **Defining models of communication**
- **Linear model of communication**
- **Interactive model of communication**
- **Transactional model of communication**

Bibliography

Kraszewski, S. and McEwan, A. (2010) *Communication Skills for Adult Nurses.* Open University Press, Maidenhead.

McCabe, C. and Timmins, F. (2006) *Communication Skills for Nursing Practice.* Palgrave MacMillan, Basingstoke.

Schramm, W. (1954) How communication works. In *The Process and Effects of Communication*, Schramm, W. (ed.), pp. 3–26. University of Illinois Press, Urbana, IL.

Shannon, C.E. and Weaver, W. (1949) *A Mathematical Model of Communication.* University of Illinois Press, Urbana, IL.

Sully, P. and Dallas, J. (2010) *Essential Communication Skills for Nursing and Midwifery.* Elsevier Mosby, Oxford.

Webb, L. (2011) *Nursing: Communication Skills in Practice.* Oxford University Press, Oxford.

Wood, J.T. (2009) *Communication in our Lives* (4th edn). Thomson-Wadsworth, Belmont, CA.

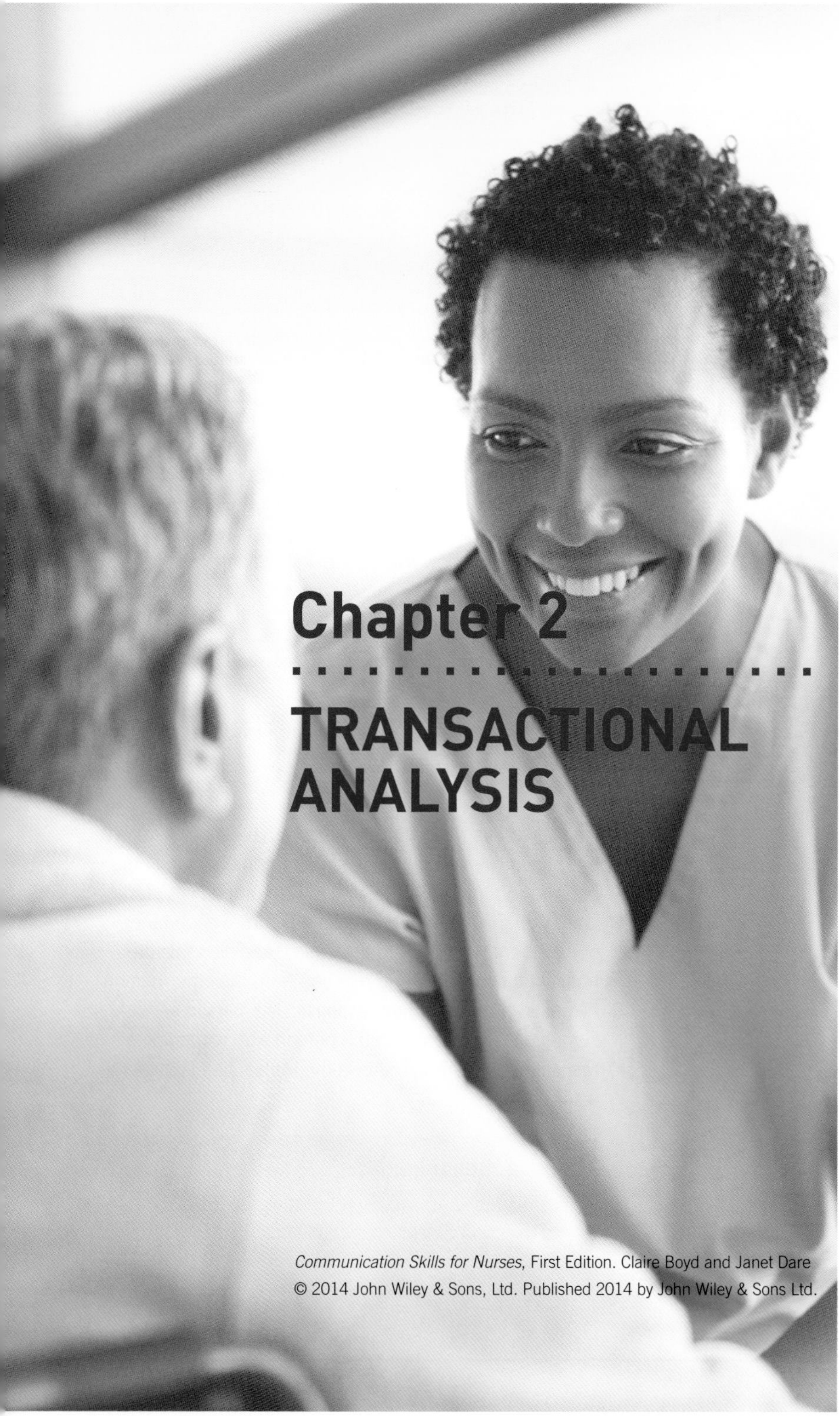

Chapter 2

TRANSACTIONAL ANALYSIS

Communication Skills for Nurses, First Edition. Claire Boyd and Janet Dare
© 2014 John Wiley & Sons, Ltd. Published 2014 by John Wiley & Sons Ltd.

LEARNING OUTCOMES

By the end of this chapter you will be able to understand how the way in which we present ourselves can influence our relationships.

Transactional analysis (or TA) was first developed by the psychiatrist Eric Berne in the late 1950s. Berne believed that our state of mind affects what happens when we interact with other people. The TA model helps to explain how people function and express their personality in their behaviour. It aims to find out what state of mind or 'ego' state started the communication process, which one responded and how this affects the relationship of the two people involved. The aim is to allow the adult ego to take control over the parent or child ego.

Berne (1964) described this state of mind as:

> a system of feelings accompanied by a related set of behaviour patterns.

He showed us that our personalities have three different ego states. We all use these states when changing our behaviour in our communication with others. His starting point was that when two people encounter each other, one of them will speak to the other. He called this the **transaction stimulus**. The reaction from the other person he called the **transaction response**. The person sending the stimulus is the **agent** and the person who responds is the **respondent**. Figure 2.1 shows the transaction stimulus in action.

GLOSSARY

Transactional analysis
An integrative approach to the theory of psychology and psychotherapy.

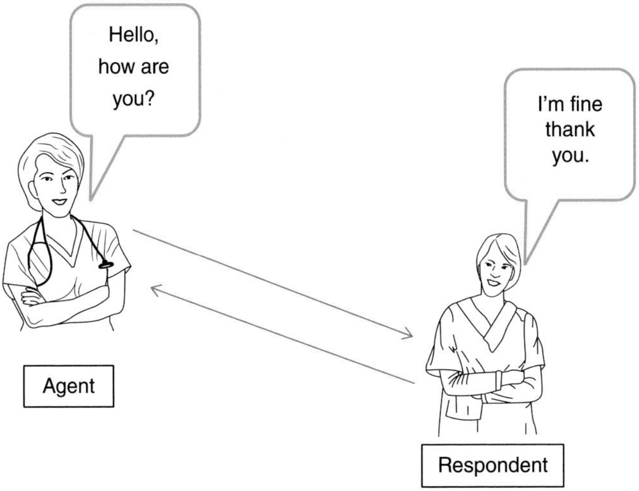

Figure 2.1 Transaction stimulus. The person on the left (agent) sends a stimulus to the person on the right. The person on the right responds (respondent). Adapted from Berne (1964). Images from http://openclipart.org.

THE EGO STATE

According to the TA model, there are three ego states that people use consistently:

P = **parent,**
A = **adult,**
C = **child.**

Transactional analysis became the method of examining the type of transaction that can be characterised by 'I do something for you, and you do something back'. Each ego state has particular verbal and non-verbal characteristics, which can be observed if you watch people. Figure 2.2 shows the three ego states.

Parent

Harris (1973) described the parent ego state as being rather like a tape recorder, in that we were conditioned by our parents or teachers, and older people. This state can be changed but it is not easy. A parent state can be caring

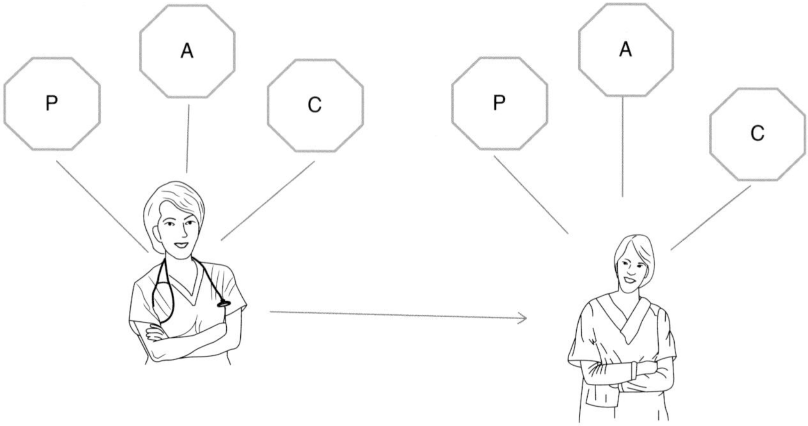

Figure 2.2 The three ego states of transactional analysis. The person on the left interacts with the person on the right. Adapted from Berne (1964). Images from http://openclipart.org.

or nurturing, such as with the reassurance that 'everything will be okay'. Or it can be judgemental and authoritarian, with the use of phrases and attitudes such as 'under no circumstances…', 'always…' and 'never forget…'. This could also include 'you will have to wait now until the end'. The parent state may use angry or impatient body language and expressions or finger-pointing gestures.

Child

Our internal reactions and feelings to external events form the child ego state. These are the seeing, hearing, feeling and emotional responses within each of us.

The state has two sides, as follows.

- **Negative**: when anger or frustration dominates reason, the child is in control. The child state has a sad expression or has temper tantrums. People in this state may say things like 'I want…', 'I don't care' or 'it's the worst day of my life!'
- **Positive**: this side of the child state is seen when a person is learning new things, exploring and being creative. They laugh, feel happy and show delight on their faces.

Like our parent state we can change the child state, but this may not be so easy to do.

Adult

Our adult ego is our ability to think and determine action for ourselves, based on received information. The adult in us begins to form at around 10 months old, and is the means by which we keep our parent and child states under control. If we are to change our parent or child state we must do so through our adult state.

Our adult ego is attentive, interested, straight-forward and uses words or phrases such as 'why?', 'what?', 'how?',' who?', 'where?', 'when?', 'how much?', 'in what way?', 'I see' and 'in my opinion…'.

Remember, when you are trying to identify ego states: words are only part of the story, it is not only what you say but how you say it and what your body language reveals. There is no general rule as to the effectiveness of any ego state in any given situation. For instance, some people get results by being dictatorial (parent to child), or by having temper tantrums (child to parent). But, for a balanced approach to life, adult to adult is generally recommended.

Transactional analysis is effectively a language within a language; a language of true meaning, feeling and motive. It can help in every situation, firstly by allowing us to understand more clearly what is going on during an interaction and, secondly, by virtue of this knowledge, by giving us a choice of what ego state to adopt, which signals to send and where to send them. This enables us to make the most of all our communications and therefore create, develop and maintain better relationships.

When we communicate we are doing so from one of our own ego states: our parent, adult or child. Our feelings at the time determine which one we use, and at any time something can trigger a shift from one state to another. When we respond, we are also doing this from one of the three states.

KINDS OF TRANSACTION

Transactions are the flow of communication. There are basically three kinds of transaction:

1. complementary (the simplest),
2. crossed,
3. ulterior (the most complex).

Complementary Transactions

At the core of Berne's theory is the rule that effective transactions (i.e. successful communications) must be complementary (see Figure 2.3). In the figure the transaction is complementary because the student nurse accepts the child ego state assigned to her by the matron and responds in the child ego state.

Crossed Transactions

In their interaction the matron and student nurse should switch between the complementary receiving and sending

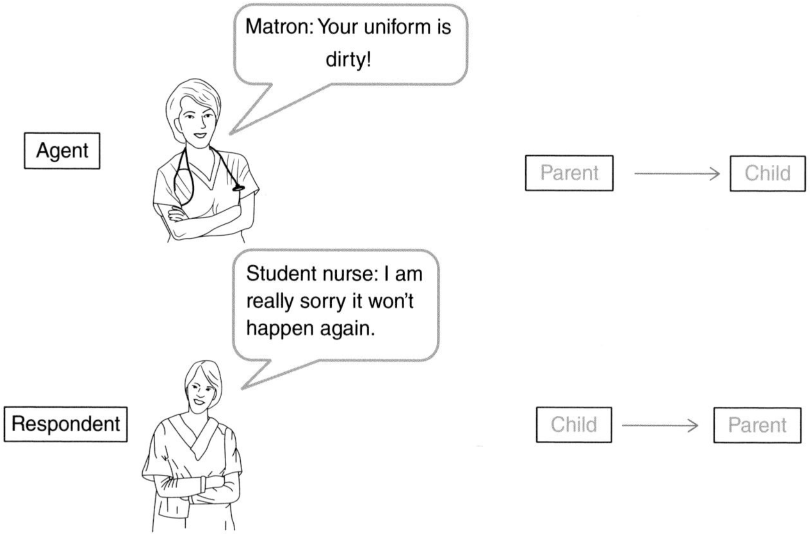

Figure 2.3 A complementary transaction. Adapted from Berne (1964). Images from http://openclipart.org.

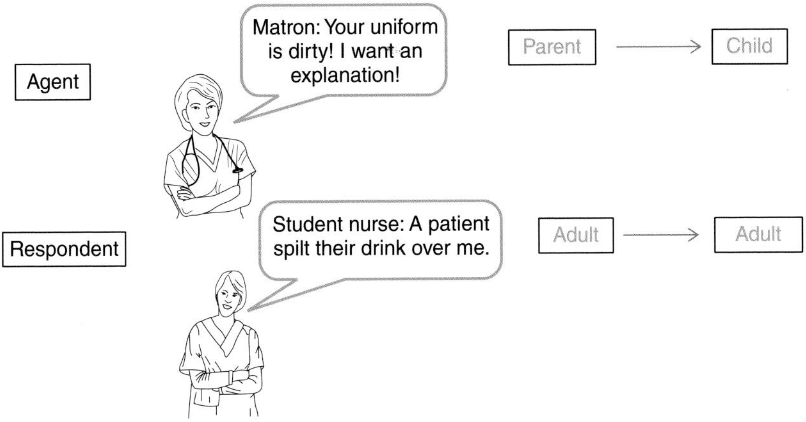

Figure 2.4 Crossed transactions. Adapted from Berne (1964). Images from http://openclipart.org.

ego states. For example, if the stimulus is parent to child, then the response should be child to parent. If this doesn't occur, then the transaction is 'crossed'; in other words, where one person has misinterpreted the ego state of the other. This is illustrated in Figure 2.4.

The transaction in Figure 2.4 is crossed because the matron, using the parent ego state, attempted to address the student nurse as a child. But the student nurse refused this ego state and responded to the matron in an adult ego state.

A further example of this can be seen in Box 2.1.

Box 2.1

A nurse is talking to an anxious patient about their operation.

Nurse: Now then Jane, there's nothing to worry about. It's only a minor operation and you will be awake and right as rain in no time.

What do you think? What age difference is there between these two people. Is Jane an adult or a child?

Now look at the same scenario but acted out in a different manner (Box 2.2).

Box 2.2

Nurse: I can see that you are very anxious about this operation. What can I do to reassure you?

Which one do you think is better? In the first scenario the nurse has taken the role of a parent figure, with an authoritative position over the patient. In the second scenario the nurse demonstrates a position of equality and speaks to the patient as one adult to another.

Now look at a different example of a tutor communicating with a student nurse in Box 2.3.

Box 2.3

Tutor: Why are you always late for your study days?

Student: I have to catch two buses to get here on a morning and it's not fair.

What states have been adopted here? The tutor has adopted a parent state and has received a child ego state from the student in return.

ACTIVITY

Activity 2.1

During an outpatient appointment a doctor tells a patient of the risks involved with continuing to smoke cigarettes. He gives a very detailed account that makes the patient very anxious, who is reluctant to follow the advice.

What states exist here?

Ulterior Transactions

Another class of transaction is the ulterior transaction. This is where an explicit social conversation occurs in parallel

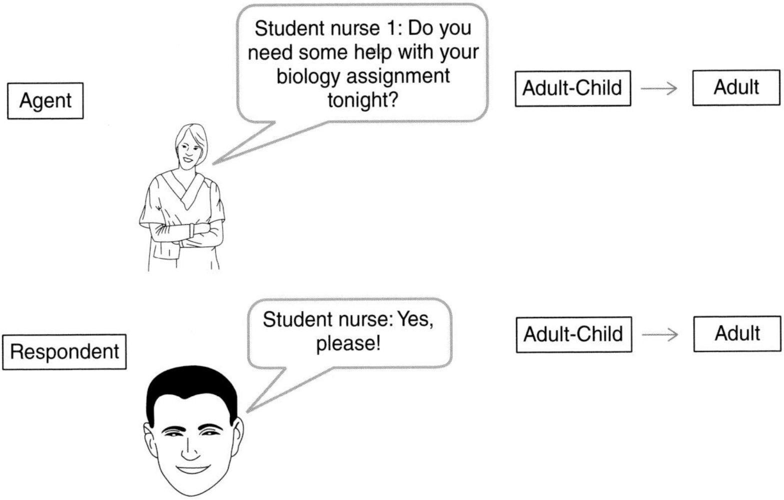

Figure 2.5 Ulterior transaction. Adapted from Berne (1964). Images from http://openclipart.org.

with an implicit psychological transaction. An example of this type of transaction can be seen in Figure 2.5.

The scenario shown in the figure is an ulterior transaction because student nurse 1 used the adult ego state to communicate adult words, but her body language actually indicated sexual intent, using the flirtatious child ego state. Student nurse 2 gave an adult response to an adult statement, but was winking and grinning: the child accepts the hidden motive.

SUMMARY OF TRANSACTIONAL ANALYSIS

Transactional analysis is a very useful communication tool because it helps us to identify the roles that people are adopting in a relationship. The student nurse will be able to read a patient's emotional state and respond appropriately.

Transactional analysis has developed significantly beyond Berne's early theories and has been explored and enhanced in many different ways by Ian Stewart and

Vann Joines. Their book *TA Today: A New Introduction to Transactional Analysis* (Stewart and Joines 1987) is widely regarded as a definitive modern interpretation.

TEST YOUR KNOWLEDGE

1. What is transactional analysis?
2. What are the three 'ego' states suggested by Eric Berne?
3. What is a crossed transaction?

KEY POINTS

- **Transactional analysis**
- **Ego states**
- **Types of transaction**

Bibliography

Berne, E. (1964) *Games People Play: The Psychology of Human Relationships.* Penguin Books, New York.

Harris, T.A. (1973) *I'm O.K., You're O.K.* Pan Books, London.

ILM Management Extra (2007) *Effective Communications.* Pergamon Flexible Learning, Oxford.

Stewart, I. and Joines, V. (1987) *TA Today; A New Introduction to Transactional Analysis* (2nd edn). Lifespace Publishing, Oxford.

Sully, P. and Dallas, J. (2010) *Essential Communication Skills for Nursing and Midwifery.* Elsevier Health Sciences, Edinburgh.

Webb, L. (2011) *Nursing: Communication Skills in Practice.* Oxford University Press, Oxford.

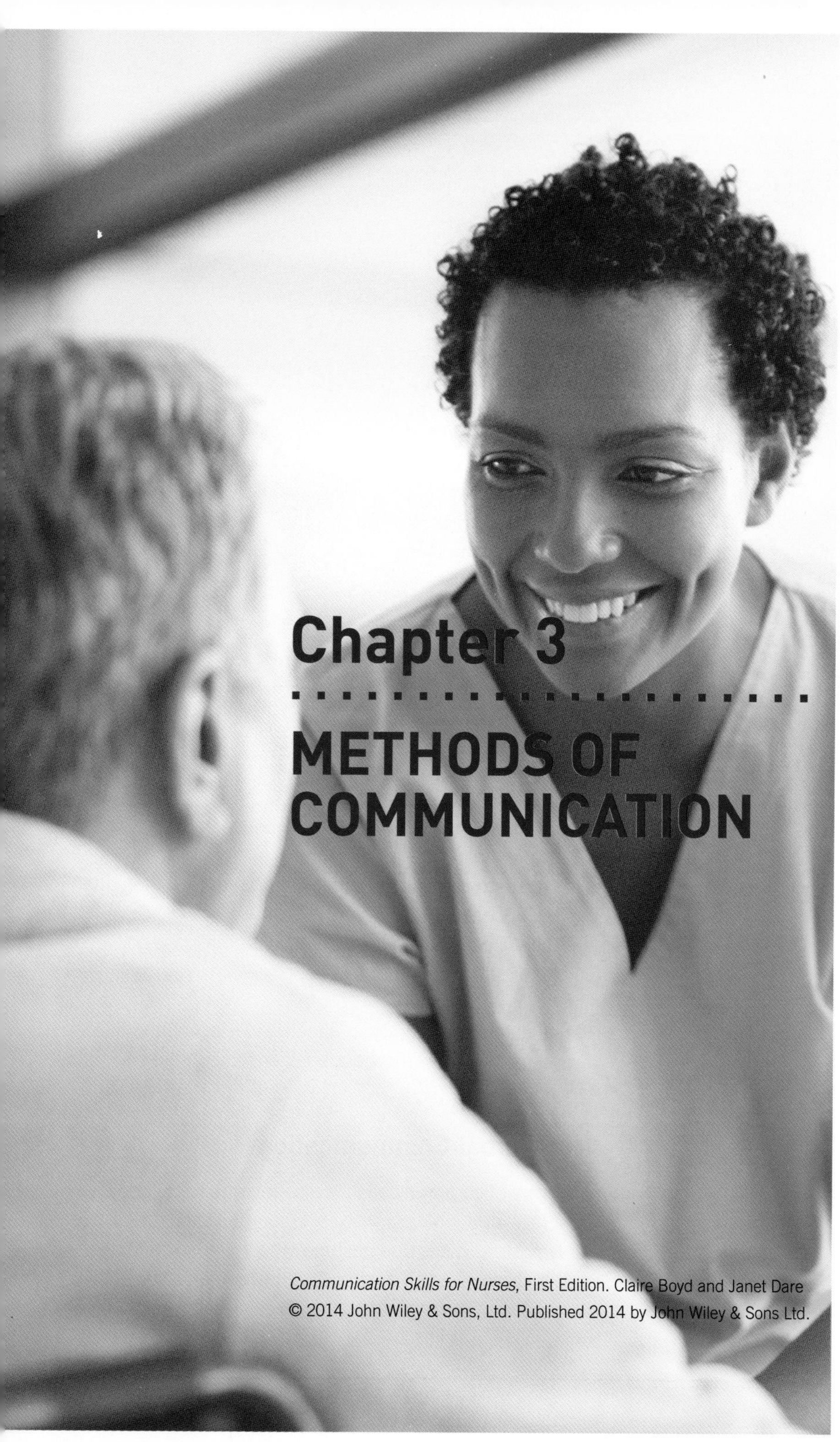

Chapter 3

METHODS OF COMMUNICATION

Communication Skills for Nurses, First Edition. Claire Boyd and Janet Dare
© 2014 John Wiley & Sons, Ltd. Published 2014 by John Wiley & Sons Ltd.

LEARNING OUTCOMES

By the end of this chapter you will have an understanding of the four main types of communication and ways of encouraging effective communication, including during the nursing handover.

TYPES OF COMMUNICATION

Good communication skills are central to the effective delivery of good-quality health care. There are four main types of communication: verbal, non-verbal, written and visual.

Verbal Communication

This type of communication includes sounds, words, language and speech and can take the form of:

- **intrapersonal** communication whereby we may process our own thoughts and actions,
- **interpersonal** communication between two individuals,
- **small-group communication** where there are more than two people involved, and
- **public communication** whereby information is conveyed to much larger groups of people.

Verbal communication is an effective way of communicating as we are able to express our emotions using spoken language.

Non-Verbal Communication

This type of communication is also referred to as 'body language' and involves physical communication, using body posture, signs and gestures, touch and expressions, and even noise, such as grunts and whimpers. Non-verbal communication often has more significance than the spoken word. Folded arms and crossed legs may be non-verbal expressions of feelings such as defensiveness. Patting and touching are forms of intimate communication and are often used to show care and compassion by the health carer. Facial expressions are used to show happiness, anger and the full range of emotions. Hands are also important communication tools, often used to express points of emphasis, while use of the feet, such as toe tapping, may express anxiety. Learning how to interpret non-verbal communication messages, such as nods, grimaces and frowns, leads to a better understanding of the patient's condition and is a skill that health care professionals should acquire.

Written Communication

This type of communication involves writing, and depends on style, vocabulary, clarity and precision of language. It is often used in the health-care setting as a means of imparting information to our patients. For example, when a patient is given a diagnosis from a health-care professional, they may not have listened to everything that was said, perhaps due to shock. Following up this information in written format, for the patient to read later, is a good way to get the information across. Figure 3.1 shows the cover of a comic-style booklet, with stickers, given to children who are due to undergo a blood transfusion. The aim of Billy Blood Drop is to remove the fear that young children may feel when undergoing this type of tissue transplant.

Written information is also used as a means of reflecting on the health care that we deliver as nurses; we can document information about the care we have given to our patients in the various care plans and assessment documents.

Visual Communication

This form of communication involves the visual display of information and includes photography, posters and all electronic forms of visual communication.

Figure 3.1 Age-appropriate patient information booklet, Billy Blood Drop, for young children having a blood transfusion. Permission to reproduce this image is granted by the National Blood Transfusion Committee. Published by NHS Blood and Transplant (NHSBT).

ACTIVITY

Activity 3.1

When and how would you use your verbal communication skills in the health-care setting? Try to think of 10 examples.

COMMUNICATION DIFFERENCES

There are many reasons for communication differences and barriers to effective communication. These will be looked at in more detail in Chapter 7. They include the following.

- **Cultural differences**: culture is about more than just language. For example, in some cultures children are not

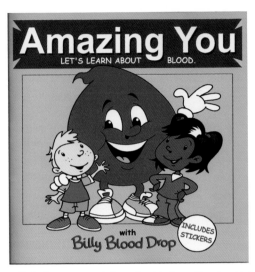

allowed to speak in the presence of certain adults, and women are not allowed to speak to men whom they do not know. Some people are brought up not to challenge authority and so may find it difficult to ask questions of a doctor, feeling that it is disrespectful to question them.

- **Language barriers**: individuals who do not understand the language being spoken can find the care setting to be isolating, frightening and even frustrating. Patients should always be involved in their own care and translators should be made available so as not to disadvantage these patients. Hospitals and other health-case settings should hold a list of interpretators (with names and contact details) in case their services are required.
- **Sensory impairment**: hearing loss can make the act of communication very difficult, often making the patient feel withdrawn and isolated. Loss of vision can make it very difficult for a patient to pick up on visual signals, perhaps hindering their ability to communicate effectively.
- **Distress** (patient unable to talk or listen due to being upset): sometimes it is appropriate to just sit with a patient and to offer human comfort.
- **Physical illness or disability** (such as confusion, stroke or learning difficulties): physical disability may result in dysphasia (difficulty with talking) and impair physical movement, making the act of non-verbal communication difficult. Confusion can include memory loss, adding to the confusion and resulting in frustration for the individual. Depending on the severity of the learning disability, understanding and the act of information processing may be affected.

WAYS TO ENCOURAGE EFFECTIVE COMMUNICATION

- **Cultural differences**: find out about the patient's background by asking a member of the family or a friend, or asking someone else from the same culture.
- **Language barriers**: smile and use friendly expressions and gestures, use pictures and repeat words to check understanding.

- **Sensory impairment**: speak clearly and listen carefully, use touch (if appropriate), remove distractions, and make sure that the patient has their usual sensory aids with them (e.g. hearing aid, glasses) and that they are working correctly/clean.
- **Distress**: comfort the patient or give the patient space if they want to be on their own.
- **Confusion**: repeat information as often as necessary, be clear and keep conversation short and simple; remain patient. There may be 'windows of opportunity' where clarity is momentarily restored and information can be given and understood.
- **Physical disability**: do not patronise; give the patient time to express themselves.
- **Learning difficulties**: judge the appropriate level of understanding, and be prepared to wait and listen carefully to responses. It may be appropriate to involve a carer in this process.

Deafblindness

People suffering from deafblindness use a variety of different communication methods, including the deafblind manual alphabet, block and British sign language.

- **Deafblind manual alphabet**: sometimes called 'finger spelling', this is conducted by spelling out words onto the deafblind person's hand. It is one of the most commonly used methods worldwide.
- **Block**: this makes use of tracing the letters of the alphabet in block capitals onto the palm of the deafblind person's hand.
- **British sign language (BSL)**: this method makes use of space and movement of the hands, face, body and head. Figure 3.2 shows the British sign language alphabet. An alternative method is Makaton, which uses signs without the grammatical structure of the BSL. An example of this is a thumbs-up signal, meaning 'good'.

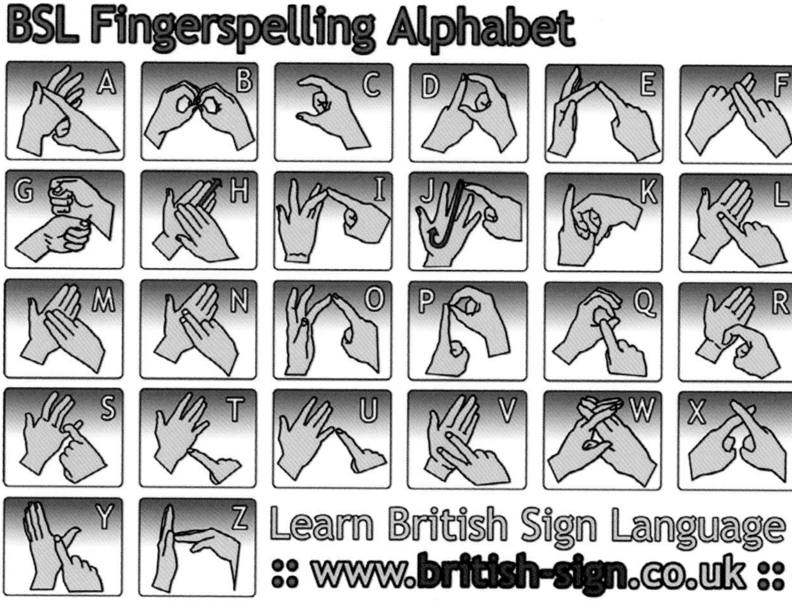

Figure 3.2 British sign language alphabet.
Source: www.british-sign.co.uk.

MEDICAL JARGON

It is important that all health-care workers communicate effectively with patients, and each other, using accessible language that can be understood by all. However, working in the care field you will have noticed the abundance of jargon and abbreviations that are used in all disciplines. I have seen jargon being used to 'show off', with the person using terminology that only a health-care professional would understand. This will only worry the patient, as they will be excluded from a discussion about their own health care and not understand what the health carer is taking about.

Below is an example of a nurse talking inappropriately to a patient.

> Hello Mrs Browne. Is it OK for me to do your *obs* before I take you to the toilet for your *EM MSU*?

What she should have said was:

> Hello Mrs Browne. The doctors have requested a urine sample. It is best if we collect an *early-morning mid-stream urine* sample. That's the middle part of the first wee of the day. So, start weeing in the toilet and then use the pot to capture the mid-stream of your wee. Remove the pot and continue weeing into the toilet. I also need to take your blood pressure and other *observations*, or vital signs. Are you happy for me to do this first, or would you like to go to the toilet first?

Of course, it is best practice to find out first what Mrs Browne prefers to call the act of micturition as it has many names, some of which are passing urine, peeing, 'spending a penny', 'going to the ladies'/little girl's room' and 'powdering my nose' just to mention a few.

Activity 3.2 lists some widely used jargon, terminology and abbreviations used in the health-care setting. See how much of it you understand.

ACTIVITY

Activity 3.2

Jargon, terminology or abbreviation	
proof of concept	PCN
efficiency savings and disinvestment	MS
let's take this discussion off-line	PE
STAT	PO

Jargon, terminology or abbreviation	
C-section	SZ
CAT/CT scan	PRN
BP	HX
FX	NKA
ABG	ICP
vitals	IHD
MRI	BSA
claudication	SOB
AF	C/O
WN	BI
TPR	CA
W/C	CL
O2	BE
PCA	BG
PC	DOA
SB	COAD
NIDDM	CSF
SS	BO
NG	DVT
GB	CP
NA	MAOIs

It's important to remember that abbreviations can be misunderstood by professionals, carers and patients. Their overuse may lead to confusion and mistakes, which can turn out to have devastating consequences. An example of this is the abbreviation DOA: in some areas this may mean 'date of admission' and in others it can mean 'dead on arrival'.

DIFFICULT PATIENT SITUATIONS

Working in the health-care profession, your role may include caring for the dying patient and comforting bereaved relatives. Grieving patients and relatives typically express a wide range of complex emotions. Traditionally it tended to be the doctor's role to inform a patient's relatives of their death, but today there is much more emphasis on multi-professional working, and it may be the nurse who delivers this news. Nurses often also act to support relatives after the news is broken by another professional. As a student nurse, you will not be expected to perform this very sensitive communication task, but you may be part of this process.

As humans we all have our own personality, and as carers we all probably will be confronted by patients who test our communication skills to the full. Figure 3.3 shows some

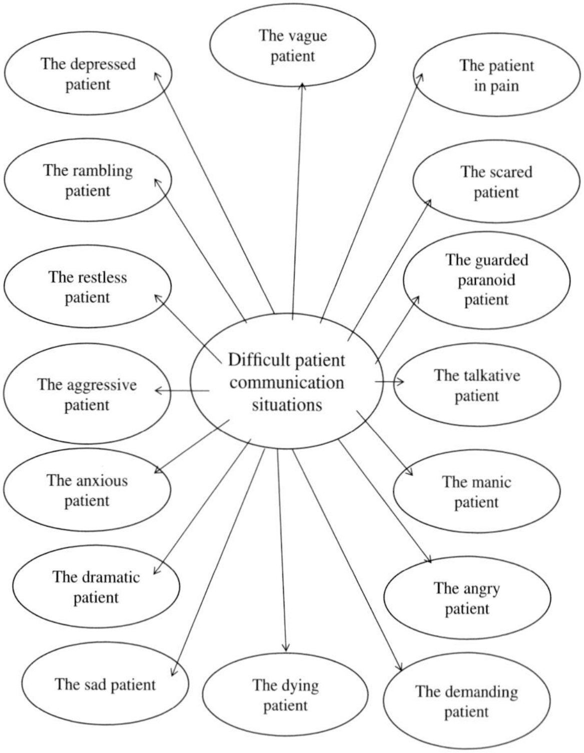

Figure 3.3 Difficult patient situations.

difficult patient situations that may impede effective nurse–patient and patient–nurse communication. It is with these patients that we will be required to utilise our care and communication skills to the full.

PAEDIATRIC NURSING COMMUNICATION

When communicating with children take into account their age and cognitive development so that you can communicate with them in an age-appropriate manner. This may mean adapting terminology to match the child's understanding. For example, when talking to a 14-year-old child about micturition, you may choose to use the word 'urine', but to a toddler it may be more appropriate to use the term 'wee wee'.

NURSING HANDOVER

The effective nursing handover is an essential component of delivering good-quality patient care. The definition of a nursing handover, also known as a nursing change of shift report, is the communication that occurs between two shifts of nurses - the specific purpose of which is to pass on information about patients under the care of the nurses (Lamond 2000). This takes place to ensure that patient care continues seamlessly, supplying the oncoming nurses with the information required to care for the patient(s) in a safe manner.

In some health-care areas this shift changeover may occur up to three times a day and have variable length. For instance, a 'full report' can last anything from 30 minutes up to an hour, or even longer. Handovers should have a clear agenda and include a safety brief. What are the priorities? Is there anything we all need to know, or any new information?

The four main types of handover are:

- verbal handover,
- tape-recorded handover,

- bedside handover,
- written handover.

Commonly, verbal handover is the selected method, whether at the bedside, nurses' station, or office. Some areas may use a pre-prepared sheet containing the patient's details, which can be shredded at the end of the shift, as with all written notes, for patient confidentiality. A 'mix-and-match' approach of both purely verbal handover without notes and written notes can also be used. For example, this can be a full report off ward with written notes followed by a verbal bedside handover.

Handovers should not just be directed towards the nurse in charge, as all nurses coming on to the shift need a handover. For example, a relative may stop you in the clinical area and ask about their relative's well-being today. It is never acceptable to say 'Sorry, he's not my patient'. If you don't know the answer to the relative's query, go and find the nurse who does. It is often at the handover that the nurse in charge formally hands over the keys for the controlled drugs cabinet (if used) to the oncoming person in charge of the shift.

ACTIVITY

Activity 3.3

Currie (2002) identified problems when conducting nursing handovers in an emergency department. What do you think these were? List four.

Currie (2002) suggested that all handovers should take the CUBAN approach:

C **confidential**: ensuring information cannot be overheard,
U **uninterrupted**: utilising a quiet area, with no distractions,
B **brief**: keeping all information brief,

A **accurate**: ensuring all information is correct and no patients are missed out,

N **named nurse**: the person who has looked after the patient should give the handover.

Box 3.1 shows examples of the type of information given during a nursing handover, by a nurse who has looked after 10 patients during her morning shift, to another nurse and a student nurse. There is a lot of good information but many details have been missed. For example, patient 1 is being discharged tomorrow: is everything ready for this discharge, such as home arrangements, prescription from pharmacy, transport, etc? Also, what are all the patients' treatment plans, observations, safety issues, etc? This is more like a handover to the whole nursing team, not to the nurse actually looking after the patients for that shift.

Also, look at all the abbreviations, which should be discouraged as much as possible. For example, do you know what MONA means? This is a treatment used for myocardial infarction (or MI), meaning that the patient has been given morphine, oxygen, nitrates (sublingual or IV) and aspirin. Read the handovers. Do they make sense to you?

QUICK TIP

You may need to look up some of the nursing terminology used in these handovers, using a nursing dictionary, or ask your Assessor in placement. For example: PU'd means passed urine, CXR is a chest X-ray and TLC means tender, loving care.

Box 3.1

Patient handovers

Patient 1

NAME: Rosemary Booker

NEXT-OF-KIN: Lives with male partner Brian Parker in Longwell Green, and 8-year-old daughter

OCCUPATION: School teacher, secondary school (history)

DOB: 15/08/1985

AGE: 29

ADMITTED: 2 days ago

PRESENTED WITH: Polyuria, dehydration, hyperventilation
Brought into emergency department via blue light with reduced consciousness
Blood glucose = 24 mmols

PROGNOSIS: Diabetic ketoacidosis

PAST MEDICAL HISTORY: Left-sided lumpectory 2004
Tonsilectomy 1992
Migraines

MEDICATION: Birth-control pill
Migraleve PRN

TREATMENT: 5% Dextrose in situ IV with sliding-scale insulin regime
Medics want blood glucose to be maintained at 10–14 mmols
Presently 10.1 mmols, receiving 3 units Actrapid insulin per hour

CARE: Nasogastric tube removed as eating and drinking. Urinary catheter also removed today, need to check she has PU'd.

FOR: U & E's, aterial blood gases and CXR today. Hoping to be discharged tomorrow.

Patient 2

NAME: Sarah Yosef, likes to be addressed as Mrs Yosef

NEXT-OF-KIN: Husband, Amir Yosef
Lives in Southmead with 8 children (ages 15–23 years old)
OCCUPATION: Housewife

DOB: 8/1/1955

AGE: 59

ADMITTED: 2 days ago, GP referral

PRESENTED WITH: Breathlessness and chest pain

PROGNOSIS: Pneumothorax, one of her daughters accidently stabbed her with a knitting needle just below clavicle

PAST MEDICAL HISTORY: Broken left femur 2012, depression

MEDICATION: Oxybutynin hydrochloride for urinary incontinence (has never sought any treatment), fluoxetine (Prozac)

TREATMENT: 28% Oxygen therapy. Due for repeat CXR. To be reviewed later today, as may be discharged. Will require TTA's to replace all her own medications.

CARE: Will require change of dressing and suture/wound care advice on discharge

Patient 3

NAME: Julie Buttons, likes to be called Buttons

NEXT-OF-KIN: Partner = Florence Thomas, Likes to be called Tom

OCCUPATION: Painter and decorator

DOB: 2/10/1993

AGE: 21

ADMITTED: Early today

PRESENTED WITH: Angioedema, rhinitis, laryngeal obstruction, hypotension, bronchospasm and tachycardia. Collapsed at home. Brought to emergency department by partner.

PROGNOSIS: Severe anaphylaxis due to eating a meal with fish

PAST MEDICAL HISTORY: Allergy to fish, asthmatic

MEDICATION: Bronchodilators, salbutamol PRN

TREATMENT: Oxygen therapy 15 Litres via non-rebreather mask. IM adrenaline, colloids for hypotension. Salbutamol infusion, and hydrocortisone

CARE: May be discharged later today. Will require allergy advice over trigger factor and advised to see GP for EpiPen

Patient 4

NAME: Pearl Hall, likes to be called Mrs Hall (widow)

NEXT-OF-KIN: Daughter, Doreen Mills (same address)

OCCUPATION: Retired domestic

DOB: 6/9/1920

AGE: 94 years

ADMITTED: 6 days ago

PRESENTED WITH: Productive cough, confusion, fever and breathlessness, chest pain

PROGNOSIS: Acute pneumonia

PAST MEDICAL HISTORY: Previous Cabg 1982, Left hip replacement 1999

MEDICATION: Aspirin 75 mg

TREATMENT: Very agitated but becoming increasingly fatigued; may be going to a HDU bed to be ventilated. On 10 day course of IV AB's

CARE: Requires 30 minutely observations – EWS. S/B Physio and requires 15 litres oxygen therapy with non-rebreather mask and constant pulse oximetry. Salbutamol nebs PRN, continue with IV fluids as necessary to keep Mrs Hall well hydrated – but check for fluid overload. On benzylpenicillin 4 grams IV QDS

Patient 5

SIDE ROOM

NAME: Paul Ryan

NEXT-OF-KIN: Wife, Zoe Ryan. Paul is presently living with his parents in London. However, girlfriend states she is NOK (lives with Paul at same address but Paul does not wish wife to know this, as they are currently on a break).

OCCUPATION: Actor

DOB: 22nd May 1985

AGE: 29 years

ADMITTED: 1/7

PRESENTED WITH: Non-productive cough, fever and breathlessness

PROGNOSIS: Left-lobe pneumonia

PAST MEDICAL HISTORY: Known alcoholic

MEDICATION: B12 injections, 3 monthly

TREATMENT: Started on acamprosate calcium for maintenance of abstinence in alcohol dependence

CARE: For CXR sometime today and then to be discharged home.
Need to obtain TTA's.
Need to vacate S/R as soon as possible for Pauleen Quartz.

Patient 6

NAME: Rebecca Mills

NEXT-OF-KIN: Mother, Mrs Kim Mills S/A

OCCUPATION: Student nurse

DOB: January 2nd, 1994

AGE: 20 years

ADMITTED: 5 days ago

PRESENTED WITH: Progressive weakness to all limbs

PROGNOSIS: Guillain–Barre syndrome secondary to herpes simplex virus

PAST MEDICAL HISTORY: No medical history but has taken illogical drugs whilst 'partying'

MEDICATION: Presently on IV immunoglobulin therapy

TREATMENT: Had CSF analysis

CARE: Presently on ECG monitoring due to autonomic instability. To be S/B neurologist and for possible transfer to neuro medical ward.

Patient 7

NAME: Xia Thomas

NEXT-OF-KIN: Husband, Brian Thomas

OCCUPATION: Retired nurse (worked in this hospital in the Renal Unit)

DOB: 1st May, 1950

AGE: 64 years

ADMITTED: Today: presently being reviewed by medic

PRESENTED WITH: Chest pain

PROGNOSIS: MI

PAST MEDICAL HISTORY: MI

MEDICATION: Atenolol 50 mg daily

TREATMENT: Transferred from emergency department and MONA implemented, Has IV access, blood gases obtained and ECG performed. Presently comfortable and sitting up in bed.

CARE:

Patient 8

NAME: Maureen Reed

NEXT-OF-KIN:

OCCUPATION:

DOB: 30th December, 1975

AGE: 38 years

ADMITTED: Last night via emergency department transferred here 5 am

PRESENTED WITH:

PROGNOSIS: Overdose of paracetamol

PAST MEDICAL HISTORY:

MEDICATION: Undertook gastric lavage and activated charcoal

TREATMENT: Observations stable. Being very sick. Very withdrawn. Not yet fully admitted. To be S/B clinical psychologist.

CARE:

Patient 9

NAME: Pauleen Quartz

NEXT-OF-KIN: Brian Quartz

OCCUPATION: Registered child minder

DOB: 23/4/1955

AGE: 59

ADMITTED: 4 days ago

PRESENTED WITH: Pyrexia and tachycardia (via GP)
Deterioration of eczema, with tender and necrotic lesions

PROGNOSIS: Eczema herpeticum, secondary to herpes simplex

PAST MEDICAL HISTORY: Eczema

MEDICATION: Topical corticosteroids, antihistimines, emollients (for eczema). Regular paracetamol

TREATMENT: Intravenous fluids. Bacterial swabs daily found *Staphylococcus aureus* (hospital-acquired infection). Also requires stool sample, as may have C-Diff: ALL precautions: May be moved to cohort ward. Will be moved to side room once vacated. Lyofoam dressings in situ for excessive exudation and topical chlorehexidine as topical antiseptic. To be prescribed IV acyclovir.

CARE:

Patient 10

SIDE ROOM

NAME: Bethan Shepard, likes to be called 'Bet'

NEXT-OF-KIN: Husband, Bert Shepard

OCCUPATION: Retired shoe factory show worker

DOB: 11th September, 1940

AGE: 75 years old

ADMITTED: 2 days ago

PRESENTED WITH: Myocardial infarction

PROGNOSIS: Not for resus. TLC only. Transferred from cardiology.

PAST MEDICAL HISTORY: Angina, left-ventricular failure. Previous MI x 2.

MEDICATION: Previous nitrates

TREATMENT: Control of pain: diamorphine, oxygen (maintenance), NG feeds.

CARE: Regular turns, and pressure relief and regular mouth and eye care. Husband remains with wife.

NOTE: Did anyone act on the safeguarding issues (vulnerable adult) of patient 2?

CRITICAL COMMUNICATIONS

Appendices 4a and 4b (in Chapter 10) show the Situation, Background, Assessment, Recommendations communications model, known as SBAR. The SBAR model can be used by any health professional to communicate clinical information about a patient's condition. This model of communication gives prompts for passing on patient information, keeping the information précised and focused.

TEST YOUR KNOWLEDGE

1. Complete the phrase: good communication skills are central to the effective delivery of _ _ _ _.
2. What are the four main types of communication?
3. List some of the difficult patient situations requiring extra care and communication skills.
4. What is the CUBAN approach to nursing handover?
5. What is SBAR?
6. Why is it important to use abbreviations with caution in the health-care setting?

KEY POINTS

- The four main types of communication
- Communication differences
- Ways of encouraging effective communication
- Medical jargon, terminology and abbreviations
- The nursing handover

Bibliography

Burnard, P. and Gill, P. (2008) *Culture, Communication and Nursing*. Pearson Education, Harlow.

Currie, J. (2002) Improving the efficiency of patient handover. *Emergency Nurse* 10(3), 24–27.

Hoban, V. (2003) How to handle a handover. *Nursing Times* 99(9), 54–55.

Lamond, D. (2000) The information content of the nurse change of shift report: a comparative study. *Journal of Advanced Nursing* 31(4), 794–804.

McCray, J. (2009) *Nursing and Multi-Professional Practice*. Sage Publications, London.

National Blood Transfusion Committee (2006) *Amazing You – Let's Learn About Blood with Billy Blood Drop*. NHS Blood and Transplant (NHSBT). www.esht.nhs.uk/EasysiteWeb/getresource.axd?AssetID=266253&type=full&servicetype=Attachment.

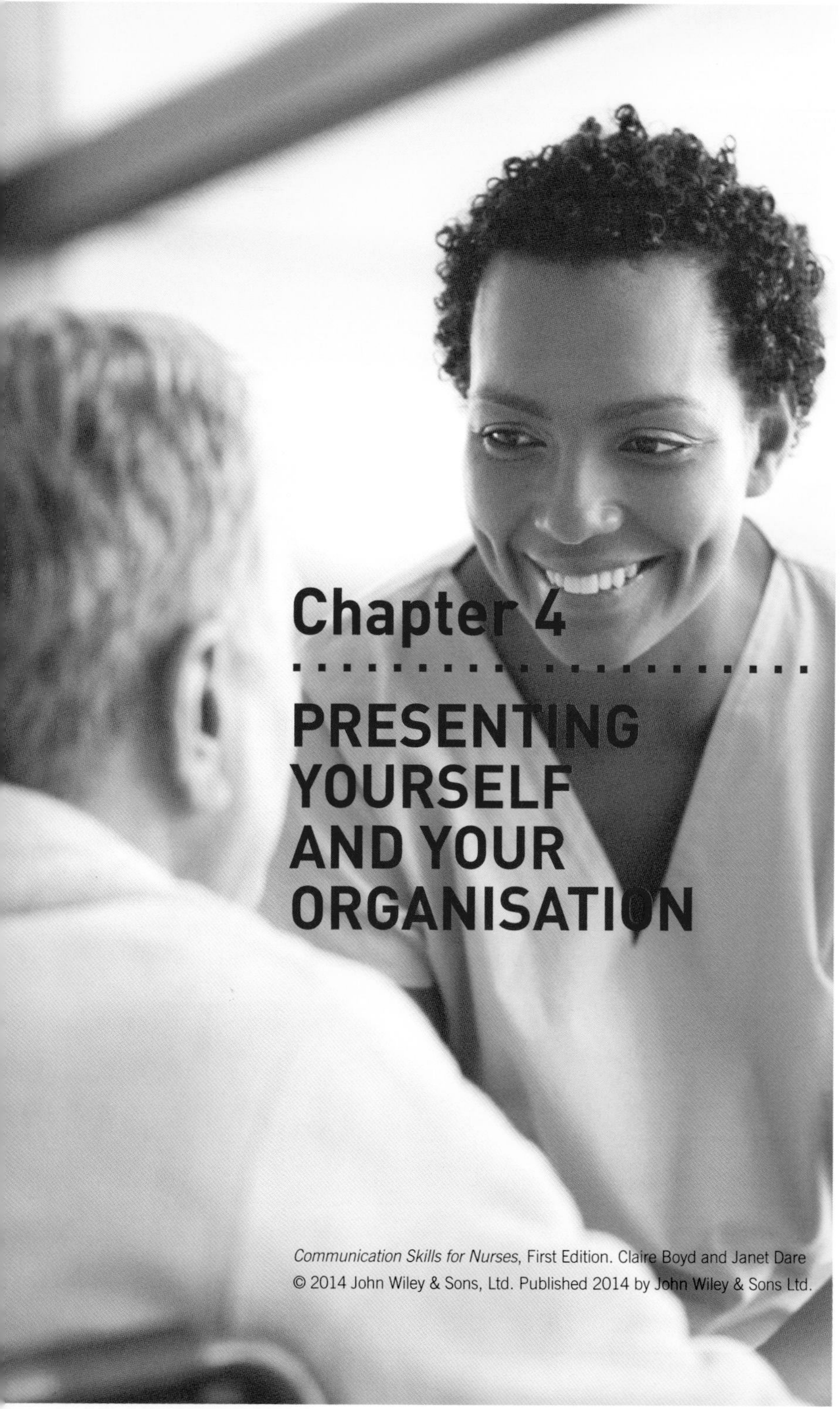

Chapter 4

PRESENTING YOURSELF AND YOUR ORGANISATION

Communication Skills for Nurses, First Edition. Claire Boyd and Janet Dare
© 2014 John Wiley & Sons, Ltd. Published 2014 by John Wiley & Sons Ltd.

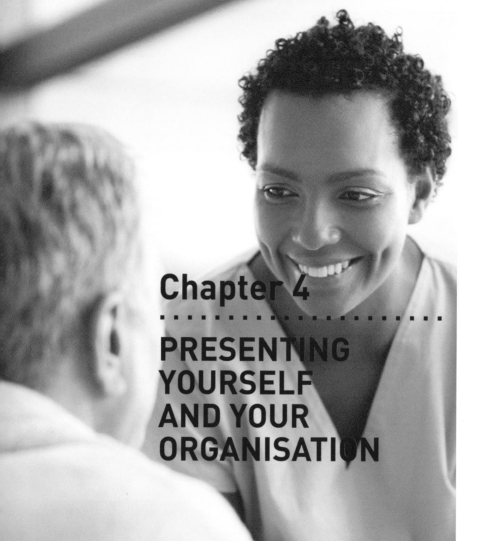

LEARNING OUTCOMES

This chapter aims to give you an understanding on the factors that contribute to customer satisfaction and the service that customers expect.

Good customer service is usually associated with the retail trade or business, but it also extends to patient care.

ACTIVITY

Activity 4.1

Write a sentence stating what you think is meant by a customer.

Patients can feel vulnerable when they are in hospital and they are in need of excellent service. The NHS Confederation, which is an independent body for the organisations that make up the modern NHS, has published a report on patient experience entitled *Feeling Better? Improving Patient Experience In Hospital* (NHS Confederation 2011). The report states that the quality of the patient experience has a direct effect on whether patients develop complications or need readmission.

ACTIVITY

Activity 4.2

What difference do you think it makes when a hospital regards the people it serves as customers rather than patients? Write down at least three ideas.

The difference between a customer and a patient is that a customer expects good service and is in a position to demand it. James Merlino, MD, Chief Experience Officer at Cleveland Clinic in the USA and President and Founder of the Association for Patient Experience, states that:

> Hospital 'customers' are very different for one important reason: they don't want to be there. The experience is scary, confusing, and they often feel as though no one understands them.

Source: Merlino, J. (2013) Why customer service matters in the healthcare industry. http://finance.yahoo.com/blogs/the-exchange/why-customer-matters-healthcare-industry-214727535.html?soc_src=copy.

In fact, the focus on the customer/patient should be the most important thing in healthcare and ensuring patient experience is also about a hospital's philosophy about the delivery of care.

A patient also has to rely on someone else to make a decision for them. A customer makes their own decisions. For example, it used to be that meals arrived on hospital wards at fixed times and there was very little choice in the food available. Patients had to have what was on offer. Now hospitals regard the patient as a customer, which obligates them to provide a wider choice of meals served at more flexible times.

WHAT IS CUSTOMER SERVICE?

The way you present yourself, how you look and how you act is important in establishing individual's trust in you. While at work you are representing the organisation for which you work and individuals you meet form judgements not only about you but about the organisation that you represent. This judgement is made in just the first few minutes of meeting someone in the workplace. This means that much of a person's lasting impression of you is based on your appearance and manner at the beginning of the interaction.

It is said that a picture is worth more than a thousand words. The first impression could be of a receptionist, who is often the first person a patient meets on entering a doctor's surgery or hospital ward. Or it could be that you are the first person a patient speaks to when they telephone your organisation.

You may have views on this and feel that making a good first impression is merely 'judging a book by its cover'. However, creating a good impression on the first meeting means that you are likely to build and maintain a good working relationship with the patient, which is good for all concerned.

ACTIVITY

Activity 4.3

This activity looks at the principles of developing good relationships. Think of an occasion when you received excellent customer service.

1. Who supplied the service?
2. What impressed you?
3. Was the service consistent or repeated?
4. What did you feel as a result?
5. What were the long- and short-term effects of the service?

First impressions are formed by each of our five senses. On first meeting, the senses contribute to the impression you get of someone in the following way:

- sight, 83%,
- smell, 3.5%,
- hearing, 11%,
- touch, 1.5%,
- taste, 1%.

HOW CAN YOU CREATE THE RIGHT IMPRESSION?

This involves three elements, as seen in Figure 4.1.

Think about how you convey messages to other individuals through your body language. For example, consider your posture: are you standing on one foot with your arms folded, not making eye contact? Think how the patient would feel if you greeted them in this manner. It may make them feel unwanted, a nuisance and that you don't care. Not everyone is full of energy early in the morning but if you are not careful then your body language will portray a lack of care. You may feel tired but yawning could be a sign that you are bored.

Appearance is also important, if your uniform is creased or stained, your shoes are dirty, or your hair flops into your eyes, what image does this portray? It suggests that you have a 'don't care' kind of attitude.

Imagine what it must look like to a patient if you are heard having a conversation about a night out with a colleague while the patient is waiting for treatment/care.

On the phone, there is nothing worse for a patient than being passed around the telephone system and repeating the same information to everyone who answers. There is nothing wrong with not having the authority to answer a person's query, but take the time to explain to your colleague what a person wants when you transfer the call.

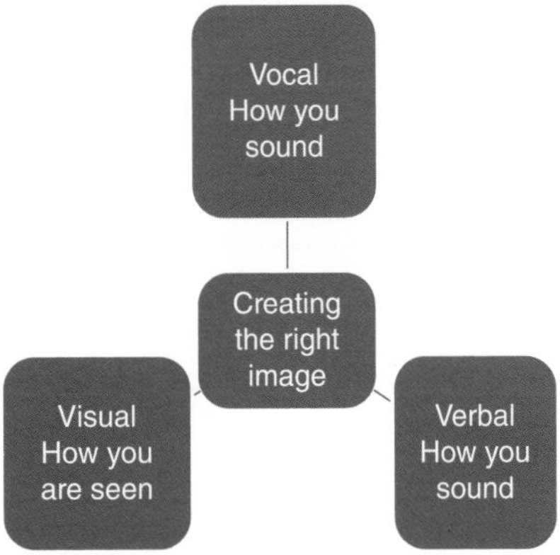

Figure 4.1 First impressions.

Finally, take a minute to look around your workplace. What impression does it make? Is the work area clean and tidy? Do the display boards have up-to-date information? Have all the equipment leads been stored safely?

QUICK TIP

Ask yourself: what can you do to create a positive impression of yourself and your organisation?

Whether you like it or not you are in control of what other people think about you. In judging you, your patients will automatically form an opinion of your organisation.

TEST YOUR KNOWLEDGE

1 What is the difference between a customer in hospital and in retail?
2 What is customer service?
3 Describe three ways in which you can create a positive impression with customers.

KEY POINTS

- Customer service
- The importance of first impressions

Bibliography

Bradley, S. (2007) *S/NVQ Customer Service. Level 2/3*. Heinemann, Oxford.

NEBS Management (2000) *Caring for the Customer*, 3rd edn. Pergamon Flexible Learning, Oxford.

NHS Confederation (2011) *Feeling Better? Improving Patient Experience in Hospital.* www.nhsconfed.org/Publications/Documents/Feeling_better_Improving_patient_experience_in_hospital_Report.pdf.

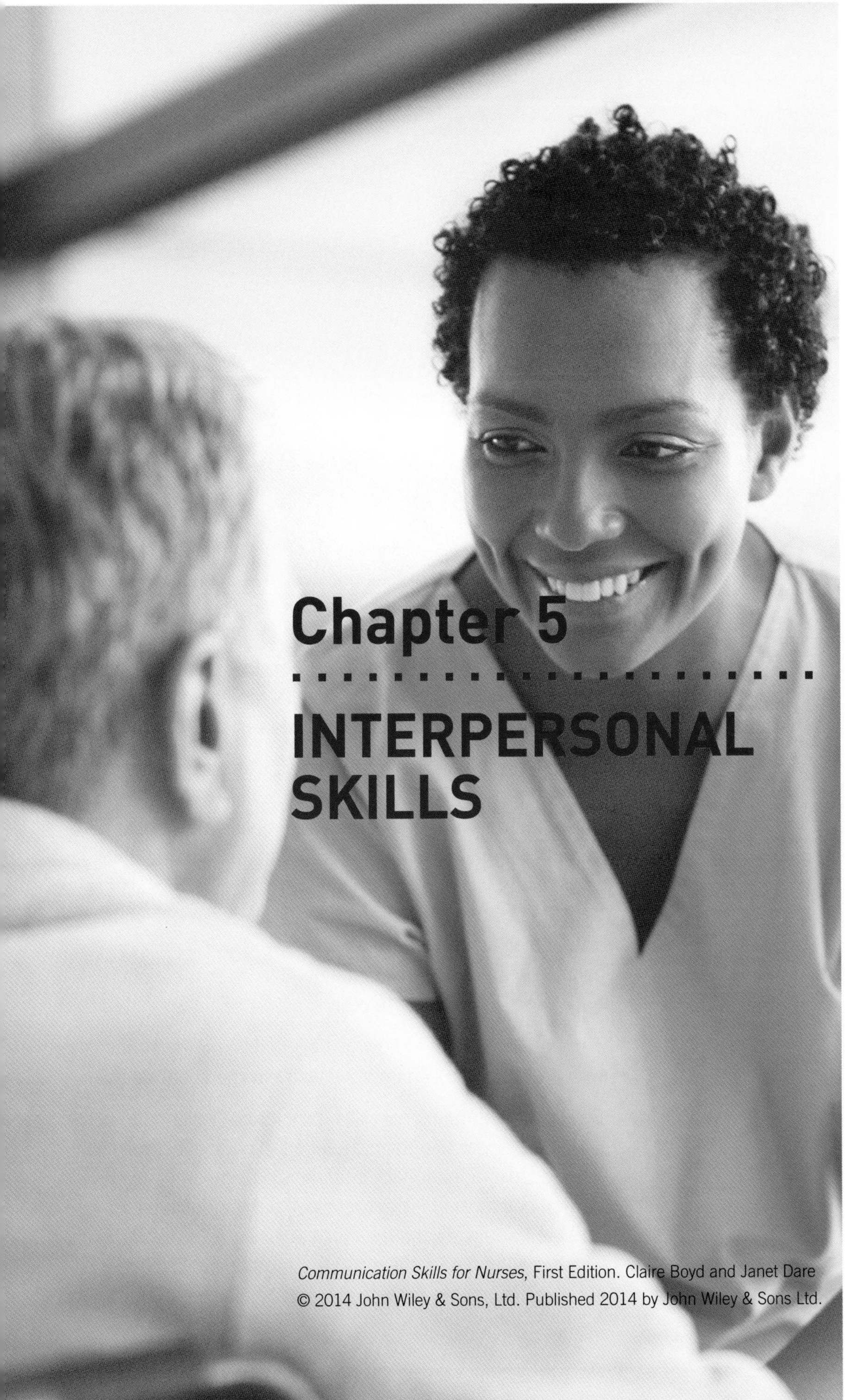

Chapter 5

INTERPERSONAL SKILLS

Communication Skills for Nurses, First Edition. Claire Boyd and Janet Dare
© 2014 John Wiley & Sons, Ltd. Published 2014 by John Wiley & Sons Ltd.

LEARNING OUTCOMES

By the end of this chapter you will be able to reflect on your own behaviour and personal style in interpersonal relationships. You will also be able to identify personal strengths and weaknesses in your interpersonal relationships.

WHAT ARE INTERPERSONAL SKILLS?

Interpersonal skills, in the health-care setting, are skills that are exhibited when nurses use evidence-based and theory-based styles of communication with their patients and colleagues. They can also be thought of as behaviours that help us to achieve an objective. People who have developed strong interpersonal skills are usually more successful in both their professional and personal lives.

Employers often seek to hire staff with 'strong interpersonal skills'; they want people who will work well in a team and be able to communicate effectively with colleagues, customers and clients. Interpersonal skills are not just important in the workplace; our personal and social lives can also benefit from better interpersonal skills. People with good interpersonal skills are usually perceived as optimistic, calm, confident and charismatic, qualities that are often endearing or appealing to others.

Through awareness of how you interact with others, and with practice, you can improve your interpersonal skills.

Developing interpersonal skills is therefore designed to help you to get all the ingredients needed to work effectively with other people. Face-to-face situations provide the context (formal or informal), objectives spell out the desirable ends, and behaviours are the means to achieve them. In situations which are not face-to-face, such as a phone call, letter or email, what you say or write represents your behaviour.

Activity 5.1

Think of someone with whom you would like to improve your interpersonal communication with in your workplace. It should be someone you interact with on a regular basis.

- Has there been any conflict with this person?
- What kind of work relationship do you have with this person?
- What positive traits do you see in this person?
- What are the negative traits you see in this person?

Interpersonal skills are all about working with other people. They include being able to support and encourage others, being able to give and receive constructive criticism as well as being able to negotiate. They are also concerned with listening to and valuing others' opinions, and being able to convey your point clearly to a group.

You will find that interpersonal skills sometimes overlap with spoken communication skills. This is because communication is crucial to good interpersonal skills.

There are just six interpersonal skills that form a process that is applicable to all situations:

- analysing the situation,
- establishing a realistic objective,
- selecting appropriate ways of behaving,
- controlling your behaviour,
- shaping other people's behaviour,
- monitoring our own and others' behaviour.

These individual skills need to be applied appropriately. For example, if you:

- are discussing how to solve a problem with a person who has more experience than you, then listening is important;

- know much more about what needs to be done to solve a problem than another person, then communicating clearly and testing the other person's understanding are higher priorities.

WHAT ARE THE INTERPERSONAL SKILLS?

1. **Effective communication** is a very important skill to have in the workplace since the main goals are to listen and comprehend what someone is saying to you. It is important to always recognise the person who is talking to you to let them know you are listening; sometimes, nodding and agreeing are ways to show that you are listening. Once the person has finished talking to you, it is important to summarise in your own words what the conversation was about, as that way the person knows you understood the conversation and that you were paying attention (this is known as *active listening* and will be explored in Chapter 8). If you have any questions about what was discussed then this is the time to ask for clarification and to repeat the conversation, making sure you understood it.
2. **Assertiveness** and assertive communication is also very important interpersonal skills in the workplace. Assertive communication skills are important, due to the fact you want to be clear, concise and to the point about what you want or need.
3. **Anger management** is also an effective interpersonal skill that is invaluable in the workplace. Everyone becomes angry about something, whether it is a bad day or someone making a mistake at work. You should not direct your anger at anyone in your workplace because this could cause intimidation and lead to workplace hostility. When you are angry take deep breaths to calm yourself down; if that does not work then just walk away. You need to learn what methods work for calming yourself down, to avoid the risk of taking your anger out on the wrong person. Workplace anger management is often taught during mandatory training when you join a large organization, but you

need to know what works for you in angry situations and how you can better control your own emotions. Knowing how and when to deal with workplace anger will better enhance the relationship between you and those you work with and will also help them to develop better anger-management skills.

4 **Conflict resolution** consists of knowing what a conflict is and how it affects you, as well as knowing the reasons why the conflict matters to you. If you are in a conflict with someone it is important to include them in your resolution while maintaining a positive attitude and acting in a civil manner toward them. Make sure they know what the conflict was and why it is important to you and also how you feel about it. Make direct compromises with the person, if possible, and ask to hear their opinion of the conflict. You should always be respectful of the other person and ask for their views on the conflict and a possible solution. When you both can agree on a resolution you should make a plan to stick to that resolution and follow it through, talking to the other person afterwards to make sure that the issue was resolved. There are conflicts in every job and everyone has an opinion about a particular subject. These may vary. Knowing how to approach a conflict and showing respect to the other person involved will help the people in your work get along and show them how they can improve their skills.

5 **Teamwork** means you can collaborate with other people and share ideas with them to arrive at a common goal. Teamwork means you are listening, cooperating with people in your workplace, communicating your thoughts and feelings and that you can come to a resolution when there is conflict. Teamwork is basically knowing you are not the only one in your workplace and that other people have ideas and feelings too, and that you all are working towards the same common outcome. Teamwork means knowing that even though some people might be different than you it is still possible to have a common goal happen by setting those differences aside. You should be able to express

your own opinions in a thoughtful and specific manner and also be able to listen to others and share ideas to help one another.

HOW CAN I DEVELOP MY INTERPERSONAL SKILLS?

There are a variety of skills that can help you to succeed in different areas of life. However, the foundations for many other skills are built on strong **interpersonal skills** because these are relevant to our **personal relationships** and **professional lives**. Without good interpersonal skills it is often more difficult to develop other important life skills.

Learn to Listen

Listening is not the same as hearing. Take time to listen carefully to what others are saying through both their verbal and non-verbal communication.

Choose Your Words

Be aware of the words you are using when talking to others. Could you be misunderstood or confuse the issue? Practise clarity and learn to seek feedback to ensure your message has been understood. Encourage others to engage in communication and use appropriate questioning to develop your understanding.

Understand Why Communication Fails

Communication is rarely perfect and can fail for a number of reasons. You will learn about the various barriers to effective communication in Chapter 7 so you can be aware of – and reduce the likelihood of – ineffective interpersonal communication and misunderstandings.

Learn to Relax

When we are nervous we tend to talk more quickly and therefore less clearly. Being tense is also evident in our body language and other non-verbal communication. Instead, try to stay calm, make eye contact and smile.

Clarify

Show an interest in the people you talk to. Ask questions and seek clarification on any points that could be easily misunderstood.

Be Positive

Try to remain positive and cheerful. People are much more likely to be drawn to you if you can maintain a positive attitude.

Empathise

Understand that other people may have different points of view. Try to see things from their perspective. You may learn something while gaining the respect and trust of others.

Understand Stress

Learn to recognise, manage and reduce stress in yourself and others. Although stress is not always bad, it can have a detrimental effect on your interpersonal communication. Learning how to recognise and manage stress, in yourself and others, is an important personal skill.

Reflect and Improve

Think about previous conversations and other interpersonal interactions; learn from your mistakes and successes. Always keep a positive attitude but realise that you can always improve your communication skills.

Negotiate

Learn how to effectively negotiate with others, paving the way for mutual respect, trust and lasting interpersonal relations.

The interpersonal skills process described above is applicable to all people and to situations anywhere, in the following ways:

- quickly analysing and assessing the situation helps us to set realistic objectives and to understand face-to-face situations;

- setting specific and realistic objectives for face-to-face encounters with people provides the context in which to make choices about how best to behave;
- by being conscious of our own behaviour in working towards the achievement of objectives we are more likely to influence other people's behaviour, thus benefiting by having an easier, and pleasant, means to achieve your objective;
- constant monitoring will provide the feedback we need to make situation-dependent adjustments.

These are just some of the potential benefits of enhanced interpersonal skills.

TEST YOUR KNOWLEDGE

1. What are interpersonal skills?
2. Identify five interpersonal skills in relation to your job role.

KEY POINTS

- **What are interpersonal skills?**
- **How to develop interpersonal skills**

Bibliography

Bach, S. and Grant, A. (2010) *Communication & Interpersonal Skills in Nursing.* Learning Matters, Exeter.

Hammick, M., Freeth, D., Copperman, J., and Goodsman, D. (2009) *Being Introprofessional.* Polity Press, London.

Webb, L. (2011) *Nursing: Communication Skills in Practice.* Oxford University Press, Oxford.

Chapter 6

TEAM WORK AND THE MULTIDISCIPLINARY TEAM

Communication Skills for Nurses, First Edition. Claire Boyd and Janet Dare
© 2014 John Wiley & Sons, Ltd. Published 2014 by John Wiley & Sons Ltd.

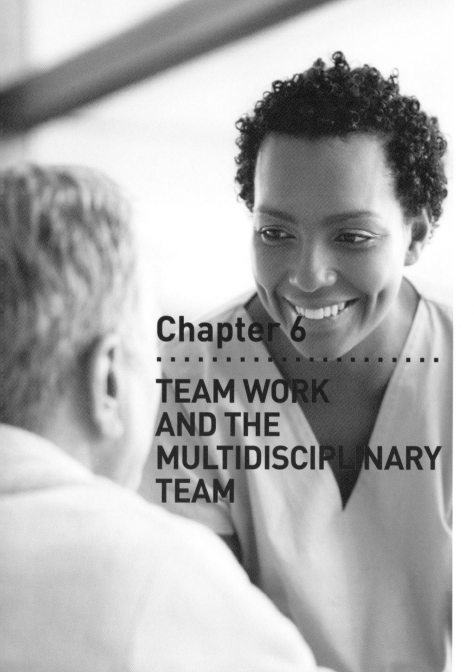

LEARNING OUTCOMES

This chapter aims to assist you to understand how a team functions and works together. You will learn how to work more effectively with colleagues, by improving your communication skills and supporting others during difficult times.

Over the years the idea of a team in the health-care setting has developed considerably and is now more complex, especially as new health-care roles have developed, such as assistant practitioner. Working well with colleagues will help you to improve the quality of care that you give to your patients.

WHAT IS A TEAM?

According to Katzenbach and Smith (1993) a team can be defined as:

> A small number of people with complementary skills who are committed to a common purpose, performance goals, and approach for which they are mutually accountable.

A good team needs to be both efficient and effective.

GLOSSARY

Efficient

Productive working with minimum wasted effort; "doing things right".

Effective

Producing the desired result; "doing the right thing".

Let us look at what makes a team effective or ineffective, and what skills are required to support good team working.

ACTIVITY

Activity 6.1

Explore the key skills and attributes required for good team working. What do you think they are?

THE MULTIDISCIPLINARY TEAM

A multidisciplinary team is a type of team that is especially common in the National Health Service (NHS), where individuals with a range of expertise and skills work together to plan, deliver and monitor health and social care with a particular patient or a group of patients.

In a hospital setting team members may include:

- social workers,
- physiotherapists,
- occupational therapists,
- dieticians,
- pharmacists.

Or, if you work in the community, they could also include:

- GPs,
- district nurses,
- chiropodist.

Dougherty and Lister (2011) state:

> Other health care specialists may also be represented on this team and can be involved in a patient's care.

Activity 6.2

Think about the individual roles of the multidisciplinary team in your work area.

How do they each contribute to patient care? Consider your own role: what can you contribute?

Think about the teams that you identified in Activity 6.2. It is likely that while some members of the team work together regularly, others are involved in a more briefer, more intermittent way. For example, a community nurse may be attached to a group of GPs and only work with other GPs occasionally for geographical reasons. In a secondary care setting, you may be discharging a patient home but require the services of a community nurse. Each person in the team needs to have an understanding of each other's role to actively participate and to feel valued.

Activity 6.3

Think about a patient who is receiving care and reflect on whether the multidisciplinary team has been effective in its actions, the patient's treatment and the overall experience.

It is often the nurse who takes the lead in co-ordinating the patient's health care by using good communication to provide a holistic care package for the patient. Owing to the increasingly complex needs of patients, teams are now expanding to include a range of health-care professionals such as a respiratory specialist nurses. However, one of the major obstacles to multidisciplinary team work is the lack of shared learning between health-care professionals; they are all educated independently.

As a student nurse you will join many different teams as you change clinical placements, and it may be difficult for you to become an effective member of a team during a short placement. One of the major challenges in a large organisation such as the NHS is the issue of working across boundaries, such as the need to encourage collaboration between primary and secondary care.

TEST YOUR KNOWLEDGE

1. What is a team?
2. What is the difference between being effective and being efficient?
3. Name one major obstacle to multidisciplinary team work.
4. List at least six people who could be in a multidisciplinary team in the health-care setting.

KEY POINTS

- **What is a team?**
- **The multidisciplinary team**
- **Interprofessional working**

Bibliography

Dougherty, L. and Lister, S. (eds) (2011) *The Royal Marsden Hospital Manual of Clinical Nursing Procedures*, 8th edn. Wiley Blackwell, Oxford.

Hammick, M., Freeth, D., Copperman, J. and Goodsman, D. (2009) *Being Introprofessional*. Polity Press, London.

Katzenbach, J.R. and Smith, D.K. (1993) *The Wisdom of Teams: Creating the High-Performance Organisation*. Harvard Business School, Boston, MA.

Sully, P. and Dallas, J. (2010) *Essential Communication Skills for Nursing and Midwifery*. Elsevier Health Sciences, Edinburgh.
Thistlewaite, J. (2012) *Values – Based Interprofessional Collaborative Practice*. Cambridge University Press, Cambridge.
Webb, L. (2011) *Nursing: Communication Skills in Practice*. Oxford University Press, Oxford.

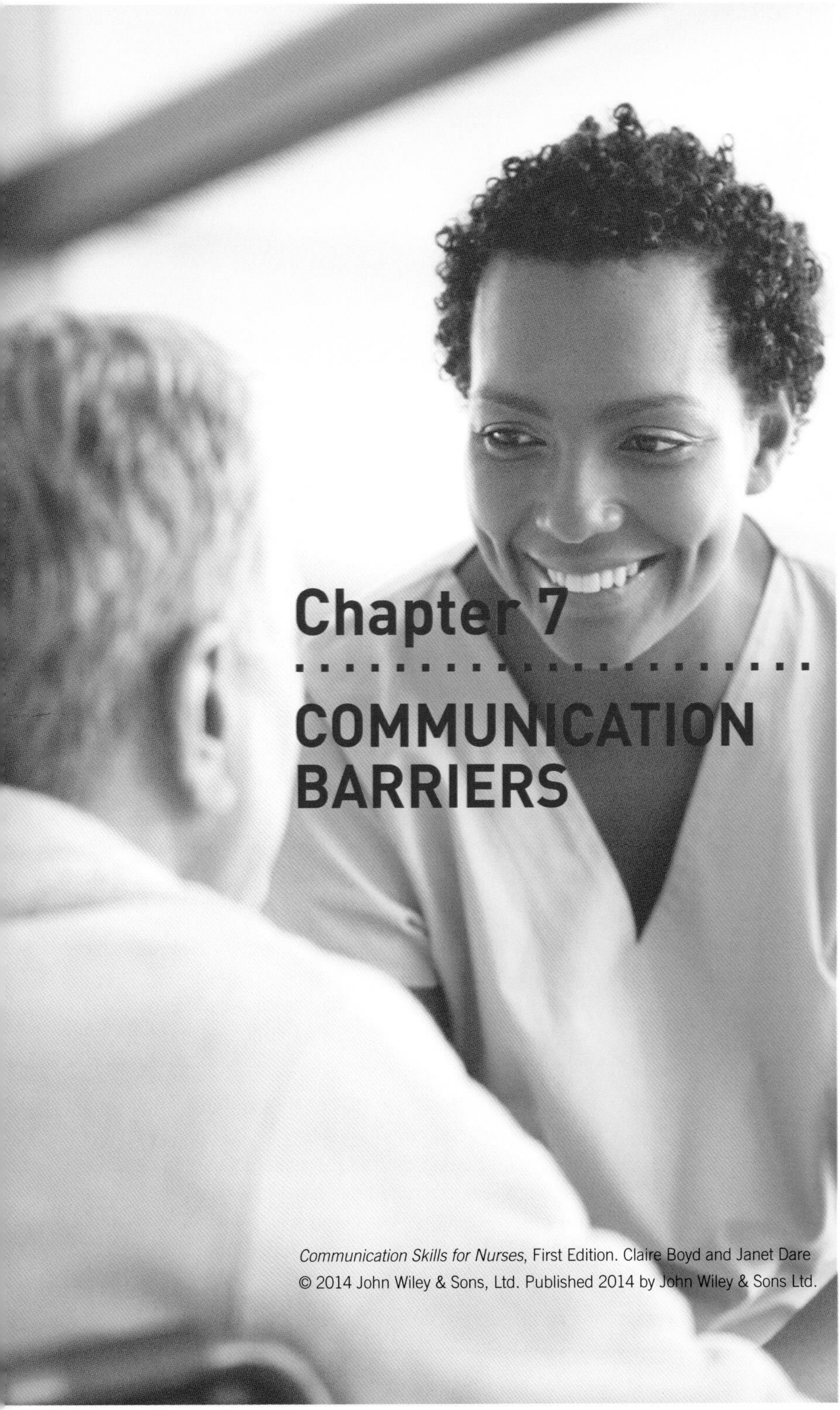

Chapter 7

COMMUNICATION BARRIERS

Communication Skills for Nurses, First Edition. Claire Boyd and Janet Dare
© 2014 John Wiley & Sons, Ltd. Published 2014 by John Wiley & Sons Ltd.

LEARNING OUTCOMES

By the end of this chapter you will be able to demonstrate knowledge and understanding of the communication barriers between nurses and their patients.

Every individual has a right to communication and we as nurses are governed by standards, policies, legislation, codes of practice and guidelines to ensure that we meet the communication needs of our patients.

How much do we take for granted with communication? Imagine how you would feel if you were unable to communicate. You may only want a cup of tea or to make a GP appointment.

Or, have you ever tried to listen to someone but not been able to concentrate because you had something else on your mind? That is because what you were thinking about was more important than what the speaker was saying. If nurses are not ready to listen then it is unlikely that a patient's message will get through.

Being able to communicate effectively is fundamental to the nursing process. A nurse has to communicate well in order to teach patients, to educate their families and collaborate with other members of the health-care team.

All nurses are likely to experience difficulty communicating with a patient at some point in their working lives (Bryan et al. 2002). In this chapter we will focus on the communication barriers between nurses and their patients.

To provide the best care for patients, a nurse must demonstrate good communication skills, providing empathy and ensuring that the patient's stay in hospital is a good experience. Nurses have the most contact time with hospital patients, and it is to the nurse that a patient may disclose any concerns, rather than to a doctor.

Have you ever witnessed a doctor's ward round and observed how patients interact with the doctor, nodding in agreement at the appropriate places? However, it is sometimes apparent from the patient's body language that they do not understand a word of what has been discussed.

THE ENVIRONMENT/PHYSICAL DISTRACTIONS

Whether you work in a hospital or a GP surgery the environment is not set up for ideal communication. Few days are ever a like, and there are times when it is very hectic. In this environment conversations or meetings are often interrupted by emergencies, or a relative or a patient with a pressing question and needing your support. Work environments can also be extremely noisy, whether it is the sound of machinery in operation, ringing telephones or general chatter.

LANGUAGE

While it is obvious that language barriers can impede communication, even people who speak the same language can experience communication barriers. The problem could be an unfamiliar accent, a speech impediment, a quiet voice, or the use of terminology that one participant in the conversation does not understand.

JARGON

Health professionals use jargon a great deal when they are communicating with their colleagues. However, it becomes a problem when they use jargon or abbreviations with an individual who does not understand what is meant. Chapter 3 looks at some of the medical jargon that is used all too frequently in the health-care setting. Another prime example of this is the use of abbreviated 'text language'. To someone who is used to sending and receiving text messages on their mobile phone this will cause no problem but to others it can be meaningless.

STEREOTYPING OR MAKING ASSUMPTIONS

This can cause major barriers to communication. Stereotyping causes us to typify a person or a group and jump to conclusions. We use our own experiences to fill in the gaps in incomplete information. This can lead to a wholly inaccurate impression of the person concerned.

ACTIVITY

Activity 7.1

Think about a time when you and a colleague have drawn two very different conclusions about a situation. Why was that?

EMOTIONS

When people are stressed or not thinking clearly, they are more apt to listen selectively or not listen at all. They can also be distracted, so they may only hear bits and pieces of your message, and take it out of context.

PAIN

Pain can be a huge barrier to communication. Have you ever broken a bone, experienced a migraine or a really bad toothache? How would you react if you had an appointment and were asked numerous questions which you did not feel well enough to answer? Imagine how a patient may feel when they are in severe pain.

ACTIVITY

Activity 7.2

Imagine that you are a patient in hospital or at a doctor's surgery and that you are unable to speak. You are about to have a dressing removed from a painful leg ulcer wound. Imagine how you would feel about your situation. Think about the specific fears you would have.

MUDDLED MESSAGES

Effective communication starts with a clear message. Contrast these two messages: "Please be here about 7:00 tomorrow morning" and "Please be here at 7:00 tomorrow morning." The one word difference makes the first message muddled and the second message clear.

Muddled messages are a barrier to communication because the sender leaves the receiver uncertain about the sender's intent. Muddled messages have many causes. The sender may be confused in his or her thinking.

NOT LISTENING/FEELINGS

Not listening is a huge communication barrier. You may be looking at someone and hearing words coming out of their mouth, but you're thinking about other things or what you will say next.

The lack of desire to participate in the communication process is a significant barrier. There is nothing more frustrating than trying to communicate with an individual who clearly does not want to do so. This often leads to a frustrating interpersonal experience that is not forgotten and which is sometimes reciprocated during subsequent encounters.

Feelings are very powerful and can prevent us from hearing properly, resulting in information being misunderstood.

CULTURE

Pease and Pease (1994) identified a range of cultural differences in the ways, such as:

- individuals may use gestures such as pointing a forefinger, which in some Asian cultures can be construed as offensive;
- invading personal space: people in some countries are less comfortable with touching than in other countries;
- some cultures greet each other with a kiss whereas others shake hands.

Doctors and nurses interact on numerous occasions during the course of a day, but often they have different perceptions of their role and responsibilities as to patient care needs. Within health care, staff come from a variety of cultural backgrounds and this highlights communication problems. For example, in some cultures people refrain from being assertive and it can be difficult for nurses from some cultures to speak up if they see something wrong.

PEOPLE WITH DISABILITIES

Communication barriers may be a problem for people with disabilities, owing to the nature of the disability. Groups who are particularly vulnerable can include:

- older people,
- children,
- people with mental health problems,
- people with learning difficulties,
- physically disabled people,
- people with sensory deficits.

NOTE: A blind person may not start a conversation with a stranger whom they cannot see.

Up to 90% of people with a learning disability have communication difficulties. This may be due to cerebral impairment leading to problems comprehending and processing information, sensory difficulties (hearing and vision), or problems in understanding social interaction, such as autism. It may also be that others do not listen or value what they are trying to say.

ACTIVITY

Activity 7.3

Tie a blindfold around your head and sit still for about 5 minutes. See how long you think 5 minutes is. Now cover your ears and do the same.

Ask a colleague to give you a drink without telling you. How did you feel?

How do you think you can help the patient to feel safe such situations?

To help consolidate and extend your understanding, try the following learning activity.

1 Find out which communication aids are available for use in your area of care. Suggestions include hearing aids, glasses, British two-handed finger spelling alphabet, sign-supported systems such as Makaton or Signalong, alphabet for names and places, photos and symbols, talking mats (for people with communication problems), high-tech aids such as Lightwriter or Stroke Talk (Connect, a communication resource for hospital care) and pictographic communication resources such as E-TRAN.

2 Familiarise yourself with their uses, and consider whether you think they are adequate for the communication needs in your area.
3 Make notes on your findings.

TEST YOUR KNOWLEDGE

Many communication barriers can be encountered while working in a health-care setting.

1 Identify three potential barriers to communication that arise at work.
2 Think about how each barrier makes communication difficult.
3 Think of ways to overcome these barriers.

KEY POINTS

- **Communication barriers**
- **Recognising the impact of disability in your care giving**

Bibliography

Bach, S. and Grant, A. (2010) *Communication & Interpersonal Skills in Nursing*. Learning Matters, Exeter.

Bryan, K., Axelrod, L., Maxim, J., Bell, L. and Jordan, L. (2002) Working with older people with communication difficulties: an evaluation of care worker training. *Aging and Mental Health* 6(3), 248–254.

ILM Management Extra (2007) *Effective Communications*. Pergamon Flexible Learning, Oxford.

Kraszewski, S. and McEwan, A. (2010) *Communication Skills for Adult Nurses*. Open University Press, Maidenhead.

Matthews, A. and Whelan, J. (1993) *In Charge of the Ward*. Blackwell Science, Oxford.

McCabe, C. and Timmins, F. (2006) *Communication Skills for Nursing Practice*. Palgrave MacMillan, Basingstoke.

Nebs Management Development Series (2007) *Communication in Management*, 3rd edn. Pergamon Flexible Learning, Oxford.

Pease, A. and Pease, B. (1994) *The Definitive Book of Body Language*. Orion Books, London.
Webb, L. (2011) *Nursing: Communication Skills in Practice*. Oxford University Press, Oxford.

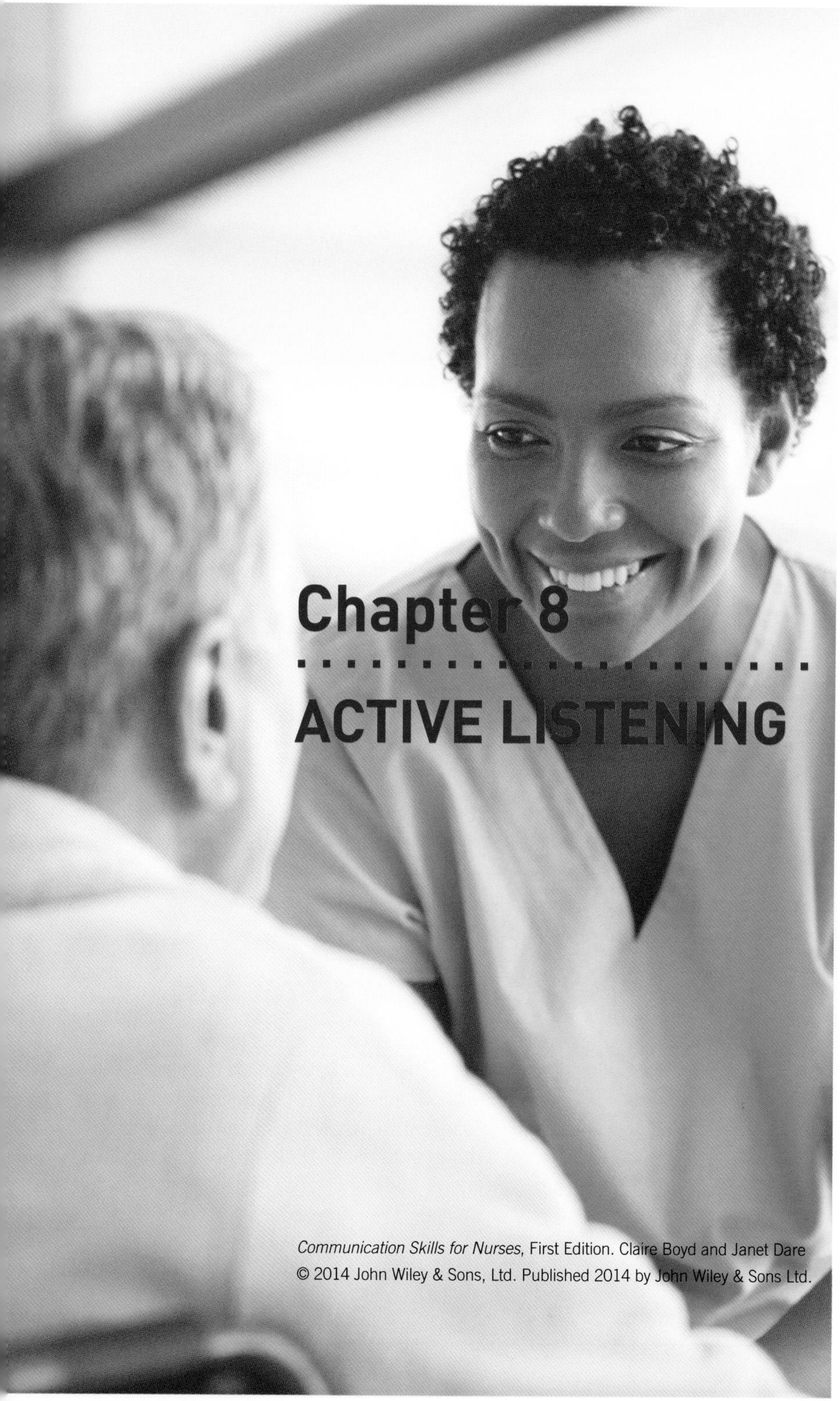

Chapter 8

ACTIVE LISTENING

Communication Skills for Nurses, First Edition. Claire Boyd and Janet Dare
© 2014 John Wiley & Sons, Ltd. Published 2014 by John Wiley & Sons Ltd.

LEARNING OUTCOMES

By the end of this chapter, you will have an understanding of active and effective listening skills and of the human factors concept.

Anyone working in health care should possess good listening skills and specifically good **active listening** skills. For instance, a patient asks you: "Some months have 31 days, some have 30 days but how many have 28 days?" The answer is that *all* months have 28 days.

How many of you actually took on board what you were being asked? Be honest, how many of us listen intently to everyone we converse with? When you are at university listening to a lecture, how often do you 'zone out' by daydreaming or simply looking out of the window? We are obviously not listening attentively. Then, you hear your lecturer state that at the end of today's lecture you will be tested and these marks will go towards your final grades! Now you've sitting up and taking note!

During times of conflict we often may have started to formulate a response during a conversation before the speaker has completed their sentence and therefore may not have listened to what was actually being said. This is where misunderstandings may occur.

WHAT IS ACTIVE LISTENING?

Active listening is a structured form of listening and responding that focuses the attention on the speaker. It is a communication technique that requires the listener to re-state or paraphrase what they have heard, in their own words. This acts to check understanding, so that the speaker knows that the listener has really understood what has been said. If not, the speaker can explain again. This minimises the chances of assumption or interpretation and of mistakes being made. The listener does not have to agree with the speaker. The benefits of active listening are:

- it forces people to listen attentively to others;
- it avoids misunderstandings as individuals have to confirm that they have understood what has been said;
- it helps during conflicts as solutions are more likely to be found if both parties are actively listening.

ACTIVE LISTENING SKILLS EXAMPLES

Look at the two conversations below. Which do you think is an example of good active listening skills, and which is a poor example?

Example 1

Patient: I am hungry. Please feed me this ice cream.

Nurse: You sound like you need something to eat. I bet you could feed yourself the ice cream if you tried.

Patient: I can't – feed me!

Nurse: Let me give you this special spoon, which you may find helpful to feed yourself and I'll be right here if you need me.

Example 2

Patient: I am hungry. Please feed me this ice cream.

Nurse: You'll need to start eating your ice cream soon, or it'll melt.

Patient: Feed me!

Nurse: Would you like a cup of tea?

Answer

Well obviously in example 1 the nurse used her active listening skills and offered encouragement, but showed the patient she had heard what was being said. In example 2 the nurse seemed to ignore the patient completely! Of course, not all examples in the real world are quite so clear cut.

ACTIVITY

Activity 8.1

Let's see how effective your active listening skills are. Answer Yes or No to the following questions. The more 'Yeses' you tick, the better your skills.

1. Do you maintain eye contact with the speaker?
2. Do you listen actively even if you do not agree with what the speaker is saying?
3. Do you encourage the speaker with nods and facial expressions?
4. Do you ask questions to check understanding?
5. Do you pay attention to the speaker's body language when you listen?
6. Do you concentrate hard when you listen to someone speaking?
7. Do you summarise what has been said to check your understanding?
8. Are you aware of the speaker's feelings when they speak?
9. Do you allow the speaker to finish talking and not interrupt?
10. Do you mentally prepare a response while the speaker is still talking?

HOW TO PERFORM EFFECTIVE ACTIVE LISTENING SKILLS

Active listening may have to be learned and practised to become perfect. The active listener should:

- face the speaker;
- maintain eye contact;

- respond appropriately to show your understanding: validating statements and making statements of support;
- try to minimise external distractions: give the speaker your full attention;
- try to minimise internal distractions: listen to what is being said and stay focused;
- focus solely on the person speaking to you and what they are saying;
- avoid letting the speaker know how you handled a similar situation;
- show good manners: even if the speaker is making a complaint about you, allow them to finish before defending yourself;
- engage yourself: ask questions for clarification;
- keep an open mind.

BARRIERS TO LISTENING

There are many things that may hinder listening skills, which were explored in Chapter 7, such as:

1. your own bias or prejudices;
2. language differences or accents;
3. noise and external distractions;
4. worry, fear, anger: not being able to focus;
5. lack of attention span (due to tiredness, etc.).

Active learning can be incorporated in all areas of health care and when these skills are not utilised effectively problems may occur.

IMPLEMENTING HUMAN FACTORS IN HEALTH CARE

The English poet Alexander Pope told us that 'To err is human'. In short, we all make mistakes. This is known as the human factor. In health care, human factors relate to all the factors that can influence people and their behaviour in the workplace. In the NHS, tens of thousands of patients get treated safely by dedicated health-care professionals, but an unacceptable number of patients are harmed within the health-care environment as a result of their treatment or as a consequence of their admission to hospital. Some of the common factors that can increase risk include:

- mental workload;
- distractions;
- the physical environment;
- physical demands;
- device/product design;
- process design.

Awareness of human factors in health care can help you to:

- understand why health-care staff make errors and, in particular, which 'systems factors' threaten patient safety;
- improve the safety culture of teams and organisations;
- enhance teamwork and improve communication between health-care staff;
- improve the design of health-care systems and equipment;
- identify 'what went wrong' and predict 'what could go wrong';
- appreciate how certain tools may help to lessen the likelihood of patient harm.
  (Patient Safety First 2009).

The area of communication is a prime example of where human factors can come into play. Let's look at the scenario below.

You are looking after the patient Anita Goolam, who has just been transferred to your ward. The nurse handing Anita over to your care states:

This is Mrs Anita Goolam, aged 65, who is recovering from bowel surgery. She had a section of bowel removed 3 days ago, due to a cancerous tumour. She has been stable post-op and not encountered any major problems. She now has a temporary colostomy, which is functioning. She is married, has three children and works part time as a librarian. She is a very chatty lady. She is a non-insulin-dependent diabetic. She has no medical history of note. She has been seen this morning by the stoma nurse specialist and is aware that her surgery was a result of a cancerous tumour. She has been seen by the MacMillan nurse specialist. Her observations (taken 30 minutes ago) are as follows:

Respirations: 14 breaths per minute
Oxygen saturations: 95% on air
Pulse: 65 beats per minute
Blood pressure: 120/70 mmHg
Temperature: 37.2°C
Blood glucose: 6.2 mmol/L

You then go and introduce yourself to Mrs Goolam, asking her what she likes to be called. You ask Anita how she is feeling and she mentions to you that she feels a bit light headed and slightly nauseous, with some abdominal pain. Your clinical area is short-staffed and you are very tired and feeling very stressed. You go about your business, preparing patients for surgery and performing vital sign observations on your patients, when you receive a message 3 hours later that your son has been sick at school and you need to collect him immediately to take him home. After making arrangements with the Ward Sister to go home, you quickly hand over to the nurse taking over Anita's care:

This is Mrs Anita Goolam, aged 65. She had a section of bowel removed 3 days ago. She has been stable post-op and not encountered any major problems. She now has a temporary colostomy, which is functioning. She is a non-insulin-dependent diabetic. She has no medical history of note. She has been seen this morning by the stoma nurse specialist and is aware that her surgery was a result of a cancerous tumour. She has been seen by the MacMillan nurse specialist. Her observations are as follows:

Respirations: 14 breaths per minute
Oxygen saturations: 95% on air
Pulse: 65 beats per minute
Blood pressure: 120/70 mmHg
Temperature: 37.2°C
Blood glucose: 6.2 mmol/L

The nurse taking over the care goes to see Anita and to perform another set of observations. She notices that Anita appears very pale and sweaty and very drowsy and does not wish to chat. This nurse immediately undertakes a set of observations, which are:

Respirations: 22 breaths per minute
Oxygen saturations: 90% on air
Pulse: 100 beats per minute
Blood pressure: 80/40 mmHg
Temperature: 37.3°C
Blood glucose: 5.9 mmols/L

Question: What do you think has happened here?

Answer: on exposure, Anita is found to be bleeding profusely from her surgical site, and she is in hypovolemic shock. During your hand over you should have mentioned that Anita had said that she felt a bit light headed and slightly nauseous, with some abdominal pain. *You should have addressed these issues*, no matter how busy you were. If you had also mentioned that Anita was quite chatty previously, the second nurse would have been alerted to the fact that Anita was not 'herself' by being so quiet and drowsy.

Although all human beings are fallible, communication is vital to avoid catastrophic events and for our patients to remain safe while in our care. You may have heard Anita saying that she felt nauseous and light headed, but you did nothing to investigate or alleviate her symptoms. *Did you really listen?*

TEST YOUR KNOWLEDGE

1. What is active listening?
2. What are the benefits of active listening?
3. How would you perform effective listening skills?
4. Name four things that may hinder effective listening skills.
5. Human factors: list six common factors that can increase risk to patients in the care setting.
6. Complete the phrase: Awareness of human factors in health care can help you to …?

KEY POINTS

- **Active listening skills**
- **Barriers to listening**
- **The human factor in health care**

Bibliography

Patient Safety First (2009) *The 'How to Guide' for Implementing Human Factors in Healthcare*. Patient Safety First, London.

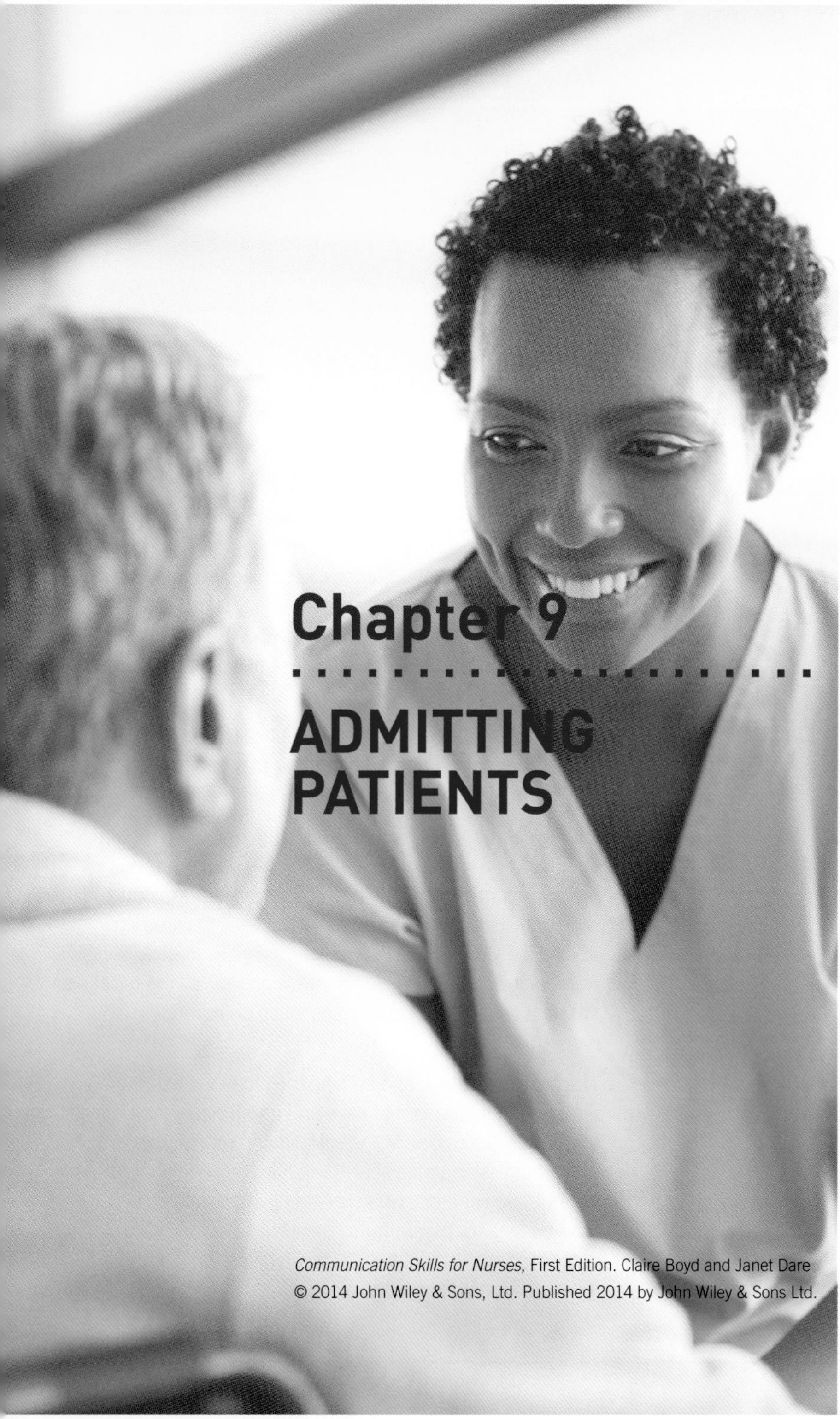

Chapter 9

ADMITTING PATIENTS

Communication Skills for Nurses, First Edition. Claire Boyd and Janet Dare
© 2014 John Wiley & Sons, Ltd. Published 2014 by John Wiley & Sons Ltd.

LEARNING OUTCOMES

By the end of this chapter you will have an understanding of the nursing process, activities of daily living and how to complete an in-patient nursing admission document.

Admitting patients on to your ward or clinical area is your opportunity to get to know a patient and should always be conducted in a warm and friendly manner. It should never be forgotten that you are representing your organisation and your conduct should be professional at all times.

It is important to gain the patient's trust and there are many strategies to assist you with this. For example, paediatric nurses may conduct the admission procedure with the small child sitting on a parent's knee. Teddy may have bandages applied in the same places as the child has theirs and injections into his arm, in a spirit of 'going through this together'.

Service users/patients in the mental health sector may feel that as they don't know you and that they can't trust you, so a lot more time may be required to build this trust.

During each admission that is conducted you are required to obtain vital information, including the patient's medical history, the medications the patient is presently taking and what activities of daily living (or ADLs) they may require assistance with. Box 9.1 shows the activities of daily living. Admission is also the time the nurse gathers all the **baseline observations**, those observations taken on admission while at rest.

The admitting nurse should take the time to talk to the patient, put the patient at ease and give the patient time to ask questions. One of the most important features of the admission process is to listen to the patient, without interruptions, while collecting information on physical health, psychological health and social health, and economic information: all having a bearing on the individual's state of health.

Box 9.1 Activities of daily living (ADL)

This is a term used in health care to refer to the self-care activities that people are able or unable to perform; ADLs are our functional status in key areas of 'living':

- maintaining a safe environment,
- communication,
- breathing,
- eating and drinking,
- elimination,
- washing and dressing,
- controlling temperature,
- mobilisation,
- working and playing,
- expressing sexuality,
- sleeping,
- death and dying.

The ADLs also incorporate biological, psychological, sociocultural, environmental and politico-economic factors.

Source: adapted from Roper (2000).

THE NURSING PROCESS

The nursing process is a dynamic and on-going cyclical process (never static) that enables the nurse to plan individualised nursing care for the patient. This planning is initiated from the information gathered from the nursing admission. Box 9.2 shows the elements of the nursing process.

Box 9.2 The nursing process

1. Assessment
2. Evaluation
3. Implementation
4. Planning
5. Diagnosis

Only by gathering the information on admission can we begin to plan care, set goals and prepare nursing actions that can then be implemented and evaluated.

Activity 9.1

There are many admission documents used in health care. Appendix 1 at the end of this chapter is one NHS Trust's document of choice, from North Bristol NHS Trust.

Below are details of a patient whose name is Hannah Jones. Work your way through the information and complete the admission documentation. Then think about the nursing care Hannah will require and what her main needs are at present (e.g. pain), and what activities of daily living Hannah will need assistance with.

Patient name: Hannah Jones
Hospital number: 789654
Date of birth: 6 June 1949
Age: you work this out!
Patient gender: Female

Patient's address: 44 Whippet Drive, Emersons Green, Bristol, BS7X 662
Prefers to be called: Ann
Admitted from: Home
Patient's phone number: 0117 987 1023
Civil status: Married
Language: English
Occupation: Retired teacher
Patient's religion: None
Patient's GP name: Dr Harris
Patient's practice: Assam Health Clinic, Emersons Green, Bristol, BS7X 661
Patient's GP phone number: 0117 321 7389

Patient's contact 1: Boris Jones
Relationship: Husband
Address: 44 Whippet Drive, Emersons Green, Bristol, BS7X 662
Phone number: 0117 987 1023
Contact at night? No
Any other information? Husband has disabilities; mobilises via wheelchair
Welfare lasting power of attorney? None

Patient's contact 2: Brian Jones
Relationship: Son
Address: Flat 7A, Hill Rise Gardens, Downend, Bristol; will presently be residing at parent's home (as above) to care for father
Phone number: mobile, 0788 899 9455 (please ring this number first)
Contact at night? Yes
Any other information: Works abroad most of the time
Welfare lasting power of attorney? None

Date of admission: Today's date
Time: 2 am
Consultant: Mrs Olah (PHO)
Diagnosis/reason for admission: Fell down stairs; fractured pelvis
Significant health history: Non-insulin dependent diabetes, osteoporosis
Where has the patient lived for the past 12 months? Home in Bristol
DNACPR: No sticker
Allergies: Penicillin
Property in safe keeping: Purse taken home by husband and son; £5.00 remains with patient

Urinalysis: pH 7 ++ Blood
Capillary blood glucose: 6.2 mmol
Weight: 102 kg
Admission observations time taken: 4:30 am
Resp rate: 18 breaths per minute
SaOz: 93% on air
Pulse: 90 beats per minute
Blood pressure: 152/80 mmHg
Temperature: 36.2°C
AVPU/GCS: Alert
EWS Track and Trigger Score:

Community care and social history: History obtained from Hannah Jones
Patient lives with: Husband
Discharge planning arrangements discussed with patient/family/other? Patient, husband and son
Hospital discharge planning leaflet given? Yes
Any dependants at home? None
Does the patient have pets? Yes: 6 cats and 1 dog
Problems with securing patient's home? None
Does the patient have keys? No, taken home by husband and son
Accommodation details: Accommodation type: Bungalow

Access details: Number of storeys = 1
Bedroom upstairs: N/A
Stair lift/lift: N/A
Number of rails on stairs: N/A
Stairs or ramp to accommodation entrance? Wheelchair access at front of bungalow
Accommodation ownership: Owned
Bathroom/toilet facilities: Bathroom/toilet upstairs? N/A
Raised toilet seat: Yes
Toilet frame: Yes
Grab rails: Yes
Bath: None, shower only
Shower: For wheelchair access, with seat

Operation/procedure: None as yet
Investigations on this admission: MRSA screen on admission. Date taken: Today. No results as yet. ECG – to be reviewed by Doctor.
Samples sent on this admission: None yet

Support at home:
- Family carer: None
- Live-in carer: None
- Home care: None
- Warden: None
- Home help: None
- Hospice/respite care: N/A
- Meals on wheels: None
- Day care: None

District nurse: None
Pharmacist: None
Key worker: None
Social worker: None
Community psychiatric nurse/ mental health care co-ordinator: None
Community matron: None
Specialist nurse: None
Community for older person: None
Other: None

Medication provision prior to admission:
Ordering prescriptions: independent
Obtaining medicines from a pharmacy: Independent
Administration of medicines: Self-administers

List of medication on admission:
Calcichew – D3 Forte calcium carbonate/colecalciterol 1.25g/10 mcg, one tablet twice a day
Alendronic acid 70 mg one tablet every 7 days
Gliclazide 80 mg daily, with breakfast

To be completed on all patients within 6 hours of admission. Please complete the following assessments for every patient:

Infection control
Venous thrombotic embolism
Falls
Pressure ulcer (skin bundle)
Malnutrition screening tool

A COMMUNICATION
Does the patient have a learning disability? No
Has the patient any specific requirement/sensory impairments? Wears glasses, remain with patient
Unable to communicate or limited communication? No
Difficulty with comprehension/understanding? No
Speech/language requirements: None
Visual requirements? None
Hearing requirements? None
Needs help with reading/writing? No

B MOBILITY

Any mobility needs that require assistance whilst in hospital? Yes, immobile at present due to fractured pelvis. To be seen by physiotherapist. Patient handling assessment chart completed

Any new problems on admission? Pain +++ on movement in bed. Action: To have regular analgesia for pain relief

Does the patient use any mobility aids/prosthesis? None

C SLEEPING

Any medication to help with sleeping? Patient requests night sedation to help with sleeping, while in hospital. Action: Medic to be informed

Any specific sleep requirements/aids that require extra resources? None

D BREATHING

Home oxygen? None

Limited mobility due to shortness of breath? None

Inhalers/nebulisers? None

Tracheostomy/laryngectomy: N/A

Does the patient smoke? One cigarette a day

Using nicotine-replacement therapy? No

Would like help to quit? Patient states she will 'give it a go'. Action: Have referred to the smoking cessation team

Lives with someone who smokes? Yes. Husband smokes approx. 20 cigs per day

E PAIN

Is the patient currently in pain (if yes, detail cause and comfort measures taken)? Yes.

Medical team aware and have prescribed analgesia, which Hannah has taken. Assistance given when repositioning in bed for comfort.

Does the patient suffer from chronic pain (if yes, detail cause and comfort measures taken)? No chronic pain.

F GENDER ISSUES RELATING TO CONDITION/TREATMENT

Has the patient any concerns about how their condition/treatment might affect their sexuality/body image or vice versa? None expressed

If female, currently menstruating? No, been through menopause

Problems with menstruation? N/A

Known to be pregnant or possibility of pregnancy (record date of last menstrual period)? N/A

Currently using oral/implanted contraception? N/A
Does the patient want or need a chaperone?

G ESSENTIAL CARE

Needs chiropody/podiatrist while in hospital? Yes, nails require cutting. Unable, due to present condition, to perform this task herself. Has been referred to chiropodist

Requires help with personal care (give details) Will require all assistance at the moment due to fractured pelvis

Does the patient have dentures? Yes, top and bottom set. Has own denture pot in bedside cabinet

H ELIMINATION

Frequency/urgency of urine? Yes, experiences urgency when wishing to void

Incontinent urine? Yes, this occurs throughout day. Wears Lady Tena incontinence pads. Has supply with her. Referral made to continence nurse advisor

Incontinent of faeces? No faecal incontinence experienced

Constipation? Yes, experiences this frequently; buys senna tablets from chemist. Will require this to be prescribed

Diarrhoea? No complaints of diarrhoea

Urethral catheter? Has urethral catheter in-situ due to injury.

Suprapubic catheter? N/A

Stoma? None

Urinary stoma? None

Nausea and/or vomiting? Has infrequent episodes when very constipated

I CULTURAL AND SPIRITUAL CARE

Actively follows a particular faith? No

Would like to see a member of the spiritual and pastoral care team or own faith leader while you are in hospital? No

Any cultural/religious practices that need help with while in hospital? No

Any faith/cultural dietary requirements? None

J ADVANCE DECISION TO REFUSE MEDICAL TREATMENT?

Does the patient have an Advance Decision to Refuse Medical Treatment (ADRMT) and/or advance care plan in place? No

Does the patient have a personal welfare lasting power of attorney? No

Does the patient need palliative care/end of life care? No

K EMOTIONAL WELL-BEING AND MENTAL HEALTH
Dementia? No
Memory loss? Patient states that 'this is nothing out of the ordinary for her age'
Emotional distress? Worried about how her husband will cope on his own
Depressed mood? None
Recent bereavement? Best friend recently 'passed away'. This was a shock and very upsetting due to the nature of her death (suicide)
Has the patient a current or history of mental health problems? None
At risk of or has currently self harmed or at risk of suicide? No
Confusion or disordered thinking? No
Acute intoxication of alcohol and drugs? No
Recreational drug use? None

L SAFEGUARDING ISSUES
Is this patient a vulnerable adult at risk of abuse or neglect by another person(s): No
Has the patient described any mistreatment? None
Are there any signs of non-accidental injury or neglect? New bruising noted on body due to fall. No signs of pressure ulcers

M MENTAL CAPACIY
May the patient lack mental capacity? No

N HEALTH PROMOTION
List health promotion leaflets/advice given and referrals made: Smoking cessation leaflet
Referral made to smoking cessation clinic
Referral made to continence nurse advisor
Referral made to chiropodist

INFORMATION

While completing this documentation, you may have come across some things you may not be familiar with, such as the meaning of some of the abbreviations.

DNACPR	this means do not resuscitate (specifically, do not attempt cardiopulmonary resuscitation)
NOK	this means next of kin

AVPU	this means Alert, Verbal, Pain or Unresponsive and is a neurological assessment (this will be explained in Chapter 10)
GCS	this is the Glasgow Coma Scale (or Score), a neurological assessment tool
EWS	this is the Early Warning Score (this will be explained in Chapter 10)

You may also have noticed that it is not just the admission documentation that needs to be completed, but also other paperwork, such as:

- infection control,
- venous thrombolic embolism,
- falls,
- pressure ulcer (skin bundles),
- malnutrition screening tool.

Box 9.3 Did you know?

- Infection control: 80% of health-care-associated urinary tract infections are related to indwelling urinary catheters (Department of Health 2007).
- Venous thrombolic embolism (VTE): it is estimated that 25 000 people are admitted to hospital die from a preventable VTE every year (Cunningham et al. 2006).
- Falls affect approximately 60 000 people every year in the UK, and result in up to 14 000 deaths (Help the Aged 2008).
- Around 65 000 patients are reported as having pressure ulcer, grade 3 and 4, in England every year (National Institute for Clinical Excellence 2005).

We will be looking at some of the documents used to communicate vital patient information in Chapter 11. Did you notice that this patient will require regular pain relief and care with her hygiene needs? Due to Hannah's lack of mobility, regular skin assessment will need to be conducted as Hannah is at high risk of developing a pressure ulcer. Also, Hannah's husband is disabled and relies on Hannah for his care, which is an issue that would need to be addressed. Their son is presently performing the carer's role.

TEST YOUR KNOWLEDGE

1. What are the elements of the nursing process?
2. Name the activities of daily living.
3. What other risk-assessment documentation will need to be completed on patient admission according to the admission documentation presented in this chapter?
4. What doe NOK mean?
5. What does GCS mean?
6. If a patient has a 'DNACPR' sticker on their notes, what does this mean?

KEY POINTS

- **How to complete a nursing admission**
- **Activities of daily living**
- **The nursing process**

Bibliography

Cunningham, M.S., White, B. and O'Donnell, J. (2006) Prevention and management of venous thromboembolism in people with cancer: a review of the evidence. *Clinical Oncology* 18(2), 145–151.

Department of Health (2006) *High Impact Intervention No 5: Urinary Catheter Care Bundle.* Department of Health, London.

Department of Health (2007) Saving Lives: A Delivery Programme to Reduce Healthcare Associated Infection Including MRSA. Department of Health, London.

Help the Aged (2008) *Falling Short.* Help the Aged, London.

National Patient Safety Agency (2007) Slips, Trips and Falls in Hospital. The Third Report from the Patient Safety Observatory. London: National Patient Safety Agency

National Institute for Clinical Excellence (2005) *The Prevention and Treatment of Pressure Ulcers.* National Institute for Clinical Excellence, London.

Roper, N., Logan, W. and Tierney, A.J. (2000) *The Roper-Logan-Tierney Model of Nursing: Based on Activities of Living.* Churchill Livingstone, London.

Siviter, B. (2008) *Student Nurse Handbook: A Survival Guide*, 2nd edn. Baillière Tindall, Edinburgh.

Appendix 1 Hospital admission documentation

North Bristol **NHS**
NHS Trust

Nursing Admission Assessment

Name (First name and Surname):	Date of admission: Time:
Hospital No:	Consultant:
Date of birth: / Age: / Female/ Male	Diagnosis/reason for admission:
Address: Post code:	Significant Health History:
Prefers to be called:	
Admitted from (please circle): Home/ nursing home / residential home / other hospital / Interhospital or trust transfer - state ward:	Where has the patient lived for the past 12 months? **Please contact the Overseas Office if the patient indicates they have lived outside the UK, as they will be asked to prove they are eligible for treatment.** Overseas Office contacted: Date: Signature:
Phone number:	
Civil status:	
Language:	
Occupation (if retired state previous occupation):	
Religion:	DNACPR: Place sticker here
GP name:	Allergies:
Practice:	Property in Safe Keeping: Place sticker here
GP phone no:	NOK/1st contact aware of admission: Informed by: Date: Time:
Contact 1.	Contact 2.
Name: Relationship: Address: Phone numbers : Contact at night? yes ☐ no ☐ Any other information? Welfare Lasting Power of Attorney?	Name: Relationship: Address: Phone numbers : Contact at night? yes ☐ no ☐ Any other information? Welfare Lasting Power of Attorney?
Signature / Name of assessing Nurse:	**Date:**

LB 17/2/11 V16.2 Frontsheet, Nursing Assessment and Discharge Documentation 1 RVJ0482 lgd

(continued)

Appendix 1 *(Continued)*

Urinalysis		Capillary Blood Glucose		Weight (Kgs)	
Admission Observations			Time Taken		

Resp Rate	SaO2	Pulse	Blood pressure	Temperature	AVPU/GCS	EWS/ Track & Trigger Score

Operations/Procedures on this admission

Operation/Procedure	Date/Time

Investigations on this admission

Investigations	Date Taken	Result
MRSA screen on admission		
NB: rescreen as per NBT policy		

Samples sent on this admission

Samples sent	Date/Time

2 LB 17/2/11 V16.2 Frontsheet, Nursing Assessment and Discharge Documentation

Patient Name	
Date of Birth	
NHS No.	

Community Care and Social History

Home Details

History obtained from?				
Patient lives with?				
Discharge planning arrangements discussed with patient/family/other?			Hospital Discharge Planning Leaflet given? (If not, state why?)	
	Tick	**Details**	**Who is caring for them while the patient is in hospital? Document action taken if further assistance required.**	
Any dependants at home?				
Does the patient have pets?				
Problems with securing patient's home?			Does the patient have keys?	

Accommodation Details

Accommodation Type	**Tick**	**Relevant Details**	**Accommodation ownership**	**Tick**	**Relevant Details**
Flat			Owned		
House			Private Rented		
Maisonette			Council Rented		
Bungalow			Housing Association		
Chalet Bungalow			NHS Institution		
Sheltered Accommodation			Private Institution		
Residential Home			**Bathroom/Toilet facilities**	**Tick**	**Relevant Details**
Nursing Home			Bathroom/toilet upstairs? (Give floor number)		
AssistedLiving			Raised toilet seat		
Rehabilitation Unit			Toilet frame		
Psychiatric Unit			Grab rails		
Custody/HMP			Bath (give details if powered bath seat)		
Hostel/Shelter			Shower (give details if level access)		
Homeless			**Further relevant information**		
Other					
Access Details	**Tick**				
Number of storeys					
Bedroom upstairs?					
Stair lift/lift					
Number of rails on stairs					
Stairs or ramp to accommodation entrance? (give details)					

Signature / Name of assessing Nurse: **Date:**

LB 17/2/11 V16.2 Frontsheet, Nursing Assessment and Discharge Documentation 3

(continued)

Appendix 1 *(Continued)*

Support at Home			
	Details/no. of visits	Name/contact Number	Services cancelled whilst in hospital? Give details, including restart notice
Family Carer			
Live-in Carer			
Home Care			
Warden			
Home Help			
Hospice/Respite Care			
Meals on Wheels			
Day Care			
District Nurse			
Pharmacist			
Key Worker			
Social Worker			
Community Psychiatric Nurse / Mental Health Care Co-ordinator			
Community Matron			
Specialist Nurse			
Community Nurse for Older Person (CNOP)			
Other			

Medication provision prior to admission				
Tick/Give details	Independent	Prompting from family/carers	Carried out by family/carers	Dossette box/ blister pack
Ordering prescriptions				
Obtaining medicines from a pharmacy				
Administration of medicines				

List of Medications on admission		

4 LB 17/2/11 V16.2 Frontsheet, Nursing Assessment and Discharge Documentation

Patient Name
Date of Birth
NHS No.

Completion Date:
Date of check (if completed in pre-op assessment):

To be completed on all patients within 6 hours of Admission.
If already completed as part of pre-op assessment, this MUST be checked by the admitting nurse when the patient is admitted.

Please complete the following risk assessments for **every** patient (*Tick box when completed)*

- **Infection Control** ☐
- **Venous Thrombotic Embolism** ☐
- **Falls** ☐
- **Pressure Ulcer (Skin Bundle)** ☐
- **Malnutrition Screening Tool** ☐

A. Communication	Yes	No	Details & Action taken	Action If 'Yes':
Does the patient have a learning disability?				**Refer to Learning disability liaison nurses** **Complete LD risk assessment**
Has the patient any specific requirements/sensory impairments				**Refer to relevant services:** • Speech & Language Therapy • Interpreter for language / British Sign Language **Complete relevant care plan e.g.** communication **If wears glasses are they with the patient? Y/N** **If wears hearing aids are they with the patient? Y/N**
Unable to communicate or limited communication				
Difficulty with comprehension/understanding				
Speech/language requirements				
Visual requirements				
Hearing requirements				
Needs help with reading/writing				
B. Mobility	**Yes**	**No**	**Details & Action taken**	**Action If 'Yes':**
Any mobility needs that require assistance whilst in hospital				**Refer to relevant services:** • Physiotherapy **Complete Patient Handling Assessment Chart** **Obtain relevant equipment** e.g. bariatric equipment
Any new problems on admission				
Does the patient use any mobility aids/prosthesis				
C. Sleeping	**Yes**	**No**	**Details & Action taken**	**Action If 'Yes':**
Any medication to help with sleeping				**Refer to relevant services:** • Medical staff **Complete relevant care plan**
Any specific sleep requirements/aids that require extra resources				

LB 17/2/11 V16.2 Frontsheet, Nursing Assessment and Discharge Documentation 5

(continued)

Appendix 1 *(Continued)*

D. Breathing	Yes	No	Details & Action taken	Action If 'Yes':
Home oxygen				**Refer to relevant services:** • Physiotherapy • ARAS team • Smoking cessation **Complete relevant care plan e.g.** tracheostomy **Brief intervention?**
Limited mobility due to shortness of breath				
Inhalers/nebulisers				
Tracheostomy/laryngectomy				
Does the patient smoke?				
Using nicotine replacement therapy?				
Would like help to quit?				
Lives with someone who smokes?				
E. Pain	**Yes**	**No**	**Details & Action taken**	**Action If 'Yes':**
Is the patient currently in pain (If yes, detail cause and comfort measures already taken)				**Refer to relevant service:** • Medical team **Complete relevant care plan e.g.** Pain management
Does the patient suffer from chronic pain (If yes, detail cause and comfort measures taken)				
F. Gender issues relating to condition / treatment	**Yes**	**No**	**Details & Action taken**	**Action If 'Yes':**
Has the patient any concerns about how their condition/treatment might affect their sexuality/body image or vice versa				**Refer to relevant services** **Carry out a pregnancy test if relevant** **Complete relevant care plans** **If pregnant, refer to the CSM team** **Refer to the Chaperone Policy if relevant**
If female, currently menstruating				
Problems with menstruation e.g. amenorrhoea/dysmenorrhoea				
Known to be pregnant or possibility of pregnancy (record date of Last Menstrual Period)				
Currently using oral/implanted contraception - Please specify				
Does the patient want or need a chaperone?				

6 LB 17/2/11 V16.2 Frontsheet, Nursing Assessment and Discharge Documentation

Patient Name	
Date of Birth	
NHS No.	

G. Essential Care	Yes	No	Details & Action taken	Action If 'Yes':
Needs chiropody/podiatrist whilst in hospital				**Refer to chiropody/podiatrist** **Refer to relevant services:** • Occupational Therapy **Complete relevant care plan:** **Start to consider discharge needs**
Requires help with personal care (give details)				
Does the patient have dentures?				
H. Elimination	**Yes**	**No**	**Details & Action taken**	**Action If 'Yes':**
Frequency/urgency of urine				**Refer to relevant services:** • Continence specialist nurse • Stoma specialist nurse • IBS specialist nurse • Medical staff **Complete relevant care plan** e.g. continence care, catheter, stoma **Complete NBT continence assessment form if continence problems**
Incontinent urine				
Incontinent faeces				
Constipation				
Diarrhoea				
Disposable pads and/or pants				
Urethral catheter (indicate if intermittent, short or long term & date of insertion)				
Suprapubic catheter				
Stoma (indicate if self caring or Requires assistance)				
Urinary stoma (indicate if self caring or requires assistance)				
Nausea and/or vomiting				
I. Cultural and Spiritual Care	**Yes**	**No**	**Details & Action taken**	**Action If 'Yes':**
Actively follows a particular faith?				**Contact the appropriate service:** • Spiritual and Pastoral Care team • Diet kitchen
Would like to see a member of the Spiritual and Pastoral Care team (Chaplaincy) or own faith leader whilst you are in hospital?				
Any cultural / religious practices that need help with whilst in hospital?				
Any faith /cultural dietary requirements?				

LB 17/2/11 V16.2 Frontsheet, Nursing Assessment and Discharge Documentation 7

(continued)

Appendix 1 *(Continued)*

J. Advance Decision to Refuse Medical Treatment (ADRMT)	Yes	No	Action If 'Yes':
Does the patient have an Advance Decision to Refuse Medical Treatment and/or advanced care plan in place?			**Refer to the ADRMT policy** **Ensure all Multidisciplinary Team are aware**
Does the patient have a Personal Welfare Lasting Power of Attorney?			**Ask patient/carer to provide documents**
Does the patient need palliative care/end of life care?			Refer to palliative care team Commence end of life care pathway

K. Emotional Well-being & Mental Health	Yes	No	Details & Action taken	Action If 'Yes':
Dementia				**Refer to/contact relevant services:** • Psychiatric liaison team • Nurse in charge if requires specialist or increased nursing care • Medical team **Complete relevant care plan** Find out details of, and contact Mental Health Care Coordinator
Memory loss				
Emotional distress				
Depressed mood				
Recent bereavement				
Has the patient a current or history of mental health problems				
At risk of or has currently self harmed or at risk of suicide				
Confusion or disordered thinking				
Acute intoxication of alcohol and drugs				
Recreational drug use				

L. Safeguarding Issues	Yes	No	Details & Action taken	Action If 'Yes':
Is this patient a vulnerable adult at risk of abuse or neglect by another person/s? (A vulnerable adult is a person over 18 who is unable to protect themselves from harm due to age, mental illness, physical disability or learning disability)				Discuss safeguarding concerns with line manager/CSM out of hours Refer to safeguarding adults policy
Has the patient described any mistreatment?				
Are there any signs of non-accidental injury or neglect e.g. dehydration, unexplained bruising, malnutrition, pressure ulcers?				

8 LB 17/2/11 V16.2 Frontsheet, Nursing Assessment and Discharge Documentation

Patient Name	
Date of Birth	
NHS No.	

M. Mental Capacity	Yes	No	Details & Action taken	Action If 'Yes':
May the patient lack mental capacity?				**Refer to the appropriate person in the Multidisciplinary team.** **See Trust Policy for Assessment of Mental Capacity and Determining Best Interests**

N. Health Promotion
List Health Promotion leaflets / advice given and referrals made:

Signature/Name of assessing Nurse:	**Date:**

LB 17/2/11 V16.2 Frontsheet, Nursing Assessment and Discharge Documentation 9

(continued)

Appendix 1 *(Continued)*

Please add any further information relating to the admission assessment below:

Area of Assessment i.e. section E	Additional Comments / Information arising from admission assessment	Date/Signature

10 LB 17/2/11 V16.2 Frontsheet, Nursing Assessment and Discharge Documentation

Patient Name	
Date of Birth	
NHS No.	

Discharge Transfer Plan

Please see admission documentation for details of care services prior to this admission

Care Support Needs

Name of person coordinating discharge:

Designation: Contact Number:

	Date / Details
Patient deemed medically stable by doctor	
Patient deemed fit and safe for discharge/transfer by MDT	
Proposed discharge/transfer date	
Patient informed of discharge/transfer	
Patient has been informed that they will be moved to the Discharge Lounge on day of discharge	
Family/carer informed of discharge/transfer	

Social services Notifications	Yes	No	Date	Name of Staff Member
Are Community Care Services likely to be needed on discharge?				
If Yes, has a Section 2 been completed?				
If discharge date has been agreed by the MDT, has a Section 5 been completed?				
Heath Needs Assessment – CM7 – completed if appropriate				
Name and contact details of allocated Social Worker				

Planned Destination on Discharge	Tick if Required	Further Details
Home with no services		
Home with support services – Home Care, District Nurse		
Alternative domiciliary accommodation i.e. family/friend's home – give address		
Intermediate Care Service - Specify		
Care home **without** nursing – specify if learning disability, EMI		
Care home **with** nursing – specify if learning disability, EMI		
Other – please specify		

Funding for future care, if appropriate (please circle)	**Self Funded**	**Social Services Funded**	**NHS Funded**
Referral for Determination of Registered Nursing Care Contribution (RNCC) when care home with nursing required	**To**.. **Date**..............................**By Whom**............................		

Has the patient been screened for Continuing Health Care? Y / N

Outcome of screening:

LB 17/2/11 V16.2 Frontsheet, Nursing Assessment and Discharge Documentation 11

(continued)

Appendix 1 *(Continued)*

Discharge Checklist					
Action Undertaken	**Date**	**Sign**	**Transportation**	**Date**	**Sign**
Patient and family/carer informed?			Transportation needs assessment		
Social Worker agreed arrangements in place for discharge			Arrangements made with relatives/carers for transportation of patient		
OT arrangements (if relevant)			Transportation ordered – (please specify)		
Physio arrangements (if relevant)			Transport type and expected arrival time on day of Discharge		
District Nurse / Health Visitor informed (if relevant)			Booking Code		
Intermediate Care confirmed (if relevant)			**Practical Arrangements**		
Home Care informed (if relevant)			Key available (please indicate access arrangements i.e. who has the key and how to contact):		
Meals on Wheels informed (if relevant)			Food and heating		
CPN/ SLT			Money and valuables returned to the patient		
Warden informed			Clothing and property returned to the patient		
GP Discharge Summary faxed on discharge			Aids and equipment given to patient (existing / new)		
If ongoing infection eg D&V, MRSA, CDiff, TB, has patient/family/carer/residence/ support services been informed			Registering with a GP if not being discharged to usual residence		
Medication and clinical care					
Advise ward pharmacist/medicine management technician of discharge date			Arrangements made for provision of new aids and equipment to go with patient (please indicate what was provided)		
TTA's written/ordered the day before discharge (NB 2 Working days required for compliance aids) (If on **WARFARIN**, ensure details on Warfarin chart fully complete)					
Patient own medication returned (if relevant) NB check dosset boxes			Any reasons that may prevent patient being moved to Discharge Lounge? (please specify)		
Discussion with patient regarding the taking of discharge medication					
Dietician (if relevant) – 5 days notice required for PEG feeds			**Follow Up**		
Dressing/equipment sent with patient			Shared care form/ District Nurse Letter		
Oxygen supplied (if relevant)			Outpatient appointment made (please specify date, time and speciality)		
Suture removal (if relevant)					
IV cannula removal (if relevant)			Patient taken off computer/admission book		
Catheter pack and letter given to patient (if catheterised on discharge); further catheter supplies arranged; handover to community team			Relevant education/leaflets given (Please specify)		
Other significant discharge information					
Signature/Name of completing Nurse:				**Date**	

12 LB 17/2/11 V16.2 Frontsheet, Nursing Assessment and Discharge Documentation

Source: North Bristol NHS Trust and University Hospitals Bristol NHS Foundation Trust. Reproduced with permission.

Chapter 10

SITUATION, BACKGROUND, ASSESSMENT, RESPONSE (SBAR)

Communication Skills for Nurses, First Edition. Claire Boyd and Janet Dare
© 2014 John Wiley & Sons, Ltd. Published 2014 by John Wiley & Sons Ltd.

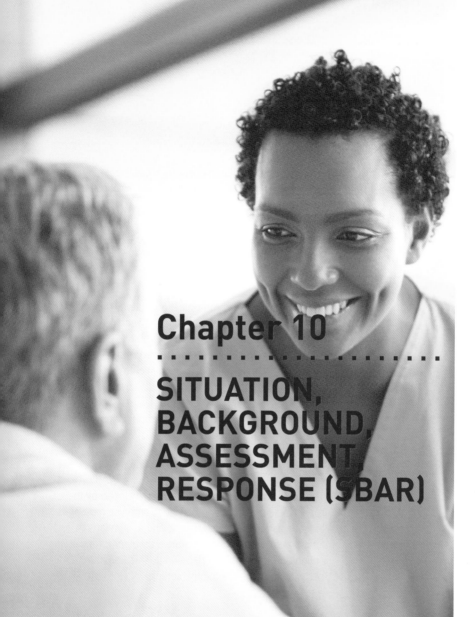

LEARNING OUTCOMES

By the end of this chapter you will have an understanding of how to use the SBAR communication tool.

How you ever wondered how you would react in an emergency situation? Would you be professionalism personified, or a quivering wreck? How would you communicate your concerns? Well, health carers are trained to use something called **critical language**, one form of which is known as the SBAR communication tool. This tool can be seen in Appendixes 4a and 4b at the end of the chapter.

The SBAR tool is a communication strategy designed to improve communication between health carers in the clinical situation, such as from nurse to clinician, from clinician to clinician, from student nurse to senior nurse, etc. It is designed to communicate our concerns regarding our patient in a succinct, concise manner (without any waffle!), and to verbalise our assessment and recommendations. In short, to communication in a clear, effective and efficient manner.

WHAT DOES SBAR MEAN?

The SBAR communication tool was developed by the US Navy Nuclear Submarine Service to organise messages in a concise and consistent way, and as a means to get attention, express concern, state a problem, propose an action and then reach a decision. SBAR was found to fit perfectly into the health-care setting.

SBAR stands for:

S **Situation:** we need to deliver the punchline in 5–10 seconds.
B **Background:** how did we get here?
A **Assessment:** what is the problem?
R **Recommendation:** what do we need to do?

Let me show you how to use the SBAR tool in a clinical situation: a patient has been admitted to hospital with a chest infection and to receive intravenous antibiotics to treat the problem. You admit the patient and take a set of observations. Plot these on the Bristol Observation Chart (see Appendix 2 at the end of the chapter). Under the Neuro Response section of the chart you will see AVPU, which is an assessment tool used in many clinical areas. This is explained in Appendix 3 at end of the chapter.

QUICK TIP

Look at the sheet regarding observations for background information. See Appendix 3 at end of the chapter.

Look at the Bristol Observation Chart shown in Appendix 2. Do you notice that each vital sign generates a score of between 0 and 3? If you tot up all these scores, known as the Early Warning Score (EWS), and if the score is 4 or more, then we need to inform a medic immediately and the nurse in charge. Simply put, EWS is a score calculated from the bedside observations, which correlates with the severity of illness. See Figure 10.1 for the nursing actions related to EWS scores.

Let's plot these scores on our observation chart:

Respiratory rate: 30 breaths per minute
Oxygen saturation (SpO_2): 93% on air
Blood pressure: 120/70 mmHg
Heart rate: 90 beats per minute
Neuro response: Alert
Temperature: 38.5°C

You will notice that two of these vital signs – the respiratory rate and the temperature – score as yellow blocks on the chart, which equates to a score of 1 each, making the patient's EWS score 2 in total.

Two hours later, you notice that the patient – Mrs Jones, aged 82 – appears to be struggling for breath. You immediately perform a set of observations and plot these on the Bristol Observation Chart.

Acting upon EWS, trigger

Score	Nursing Action
0-1	Continue
2-3	Inform nurse in charge Increase frequency of observations to hourly
≥ 4	Contact Medical team urgently via 6999 Inform nurse in charge Increase frequency of observations to half hourly

Call 2222 for cardiac arrest and peri-arrest patients

- On triggering, appropriate medical team is fast bleeped (F2 and above)
- They should review patient within 15 mins
  - Instigate treatment
  - Escalate as appropriate
- Remember, static or worsening EWS score despite treatment is a poor prognostic marker

Figure 10.1 Acting on EWS triggers.

Respiratory rate: 35 breaths per minute
Oxygen saturation (SpO_2): 89% on air
Blood pressure: 135/70 mmHg
Heart rate: 120 beats per minute
Neuro response: Verbal
Temperature: 38.2°C

We can see that our patient is deteriorating and that the *EWS score is now 7.*

ACTIVITY

Activity 10.1

This patient's EWS score is now recorded at 7: how is this made up?

Now we need to communicate this information and request an urgent review. First, I would ask a colleague to stay with my very sick patient and administer oxygen therapy via a non-rebreathe mask. Now to pass on the information. I would use my SBAR prompt sheet to keep my information clear, effective and efficient. Read this prompt sheet, which can be found in Appendix 4a.

ACTIVITY

Activity 10.2

How would you communicate the condition of your patient to a medic using the SBAR tool?

NOTES TO CONSIDER

It is important to note that you may need to convey Mrs Jones' medical history to the medic, if this is considered appropriate. For example, it was not considered necessary to state that Mrs Jones had an appendectomy 25 years ago.

It is also important to note that, as a student nurse, there is nothing to stop you from making this call after you have relayed the information to the nurse in charge. In fact, it may be more appropriate for you to do this if you have been looking after the patient and have all the patient's information.

ACTIVITY

Activity 10.3

What do the following terms mean?

Stuporous
Lethargic
Comatose

GLOSSARY

GTN

Glyceryl trinitrate. Prophylaxis and treatment for angina. Can be administered by sublingual spray, tablet format, intravenous infusion or transdermal application.

HOW NOT TO DO IT

Read the information below about a patient called Joe Smith.

Joe Smith, a 79-year-old gentleman, is experiencing chest pain which started about half an hour ago. He has known angina but has not had chest pain since his admission 2 days ago.

You are concerned about him because he is not himself and the pain does not appear to be getting any better despite giving him GTN. He did not want to eat his breakfast this morning and he refused a wash.

You carry out a set of observations. Plot these on the Bristol Observation Chart.

Respiratory rate: 28 breaths per minute
Oxygen saturation (SpO_2): 92% on air (target range 92–98%)
Heart rate: 114 beats per minute
Blood pressure: 100/60 mmHg
Neuro observations: Alert
Blood glucose: 4.2
Temperature: 37°C
Appearance is pale and clammy

Read the conversation below between a nurse and a doctor about Joe Smith. This is an example of how *not* to communicate in a critical situation.

Nurse: Hi it's me, really sorry to bother you, I know how busy you are but you know Joe Smith....

Doctor: Sorry, but who is this?

Nurse: It's me Jayne on E ward.

Doctor: OK Jayne on E ward, I am really busy as you said, so what do you want?

Nurse: It's Joe Smith. He's having a bit of chest pain and he doesn't look very good but nothing specific. He didn't want to have a wash or anything this morning and he didn't eat his breakfast.

Doctor: OK, stop there. What are his observations? His EWS?

Nurse: Oh, we are just doing them, but you really need to come and see him. I don't like the look of him.

Doctor: [sighs in frustration] Is he short of breath?

Nurse: Oh well a bit yes, it's hard to tell really.

Doctor: How long has he had the pain?

Nurse: Well I think for about half an hour.

Doctor: Look Jayne, I really don't have time for this. Call me again when you have done a set of observations and assessed the patient properly.

Nurse: But you really need... [phone is slammed down].

Well he could have at least let me finish....

Where is the urgency? The medic wants facts and figures, not waffle!

BEFORE CALLING THE CLINICIAN

Before making your call, you will need to check the following steps.

- Have I seen and assessed the patient myself before calling?

- Has the situation been discussed with the senior nurse?
- Do I know the admitting diagnosis and date of admission?
- Have I read the most recent medical notes and notes from the nurse who worked the shift before me?

MAKING THE CALL

You will need to have the following documents in front of you when speaking to the clinician:

- the patient's observation chart, to relay the most recent vital signs;
- list of current medications (prescription chart), allergies, fluid chart;
- any pathology results with dates and times that tests were conducted, and results of any previous tests for comparison;
- resuscitation status.

THE INFORMATION WE NEED TO COMMUNICATE EFFECTIVELY

So, we know to keep the communication down to brief facts, with part of the SBAR communication tool keeping to the specifics.

Situation

What is the situation you are calling about? You will need to identify yourself, your clinical area, the patient and the exact location. You will need to clearly state the problem: what is it? When did it happen or start? How severe is the problem?

Background

Information related to the situation could include the following:

- the admitting diagnosis and date of admission;
- list of current medications, allergies and IV fluids;
- most recent vital signs (using the ABCDE assessment);
- laboratory results with date and time that tests were performed, and results of previous tests for comparison;

- other clinical information: AVPU;
- resuscitation status.

Assessment

You will need to communicate your assessment of the situation, such as 'This is what I think the problem is…':

- the problem is cardiac, infection, neurological, respiratory or other;
- I don't know what the problem is but the patient is deteriorating;
- the patient is unstable and may get worse, we need to do something.

Recommendation

What is your recommendation to the clinician based on the situation and assessment:

- "I need you to come and see the patient."
- "I think we need to…."
- "Tell me what should I do next."
- "Should I contact anybody else?"
- "Should I prepare anything such as any drugs, fluids, procedure trolley"

THE FUTURE

Even as a student nurse, it is good to get to grips with the SBAR communication tool. The more you use it, the more it will become second nature. You will start off using critical language to the nurse in charge before being expected to pass on critical information about the deteriorating patient. Appendix 4b at the end of this chapter shows the full SBAR communication tool in a poster format.

TEST YOUR KNOWLEDGE

We looked at an example of how not to communicate using an example with a patient called Joe Smith. Read this information again and now, using the SBAR communication tool, communicate the information in a brief, efficient and effective manner.

KEY POINTS

- **How to use the SBAR communication tool verbally**
- **How to use the SBAR communication tool prompt sheet**
- **How to report when a patient 'triggers' on the EWS**

Bibliography

Leonard, M. (2006) The SBAR technique: improving verbal communication and teamwork in clinical care. *PONL Bulletin* 2(1).

Leonard, M., Graham, S. and Bonacum, D. (2004) The human factor: the critical importance of teamwork and communication in providing self care. *Quality & Safety in Heath Care* 13, i85–i90.

Leonard, M., Bonacum, D. and Taggart, B. (2006) *Using SBAR to Improve Communication Between Caregivers.* Institute for Healthcare Improvement, London.

Maison, D. (2006) The interdisciplinary team perspective. Effective communications are more important than ever, a physician's perspective. *Home Healthcare Nurse*, 24(3), 133–190.

Nunes, J. (2005) Patient safety leadership fellowship learnings help put theory into practice. *A Newsletter from the National Patient Safety Foundation* 8(3).

Whittington, J. and Nagamine, J. (2006) *SBAR: Application and Critical Success Factors of Implementation.* Institute for Healthcare Improvement, London.

Appendix 2 The Bristol Observation Chart

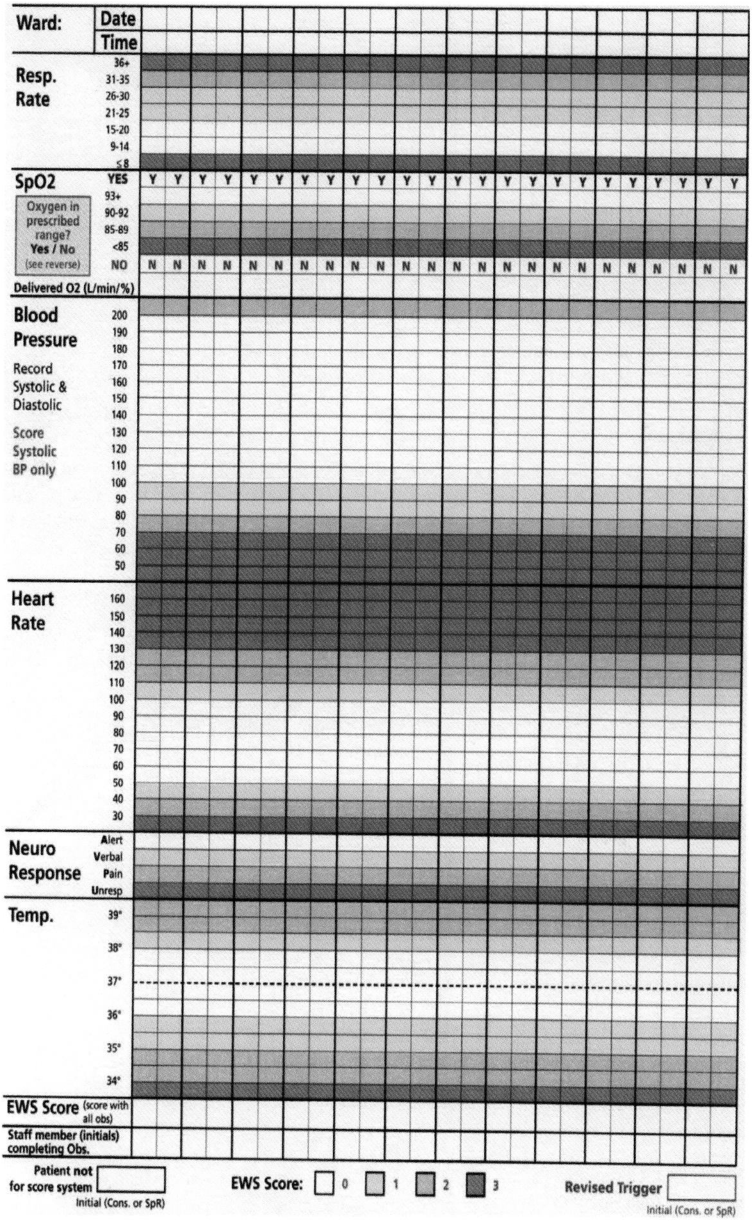

Source: North Bristol NHS Trust and University Hospitals Bristol NHS Foundation Trust. Reproduced with permission.

Appendix 3 Observation information sheet

Respirations

Healthy adults	14–20 breaths per minute
Adolescents	18–22 breaths per minute
Children	22–28 breaths per minute
Infants	30 or more breaths per minute

Oxygen saturations

These should be in the prescribed range, as seen on the prescription chart.

Symptoms of low oxygen levels in the blood (hypoxaemia)

Breathlessness, agitation, confusion, tachycardia, tachypnoea, physical tiredness, increased work of breathing, increased or decreased ventilation.

Symptoms of high levels of carbon dioxide in the blood (hypercapnoea)

Drowsiness (reduced AVPU; see below), headaches, respiratory distress, flushed face, warm peripheries, full and bounding pulse, confusion, muscle twitching, convulsions, coma.

Blood pressure

Normal range for an adult is usually considered to be from 100/60 to 140/90 mmHg. The first figure is known as the 'systolic' reading and the second figure is the 'diastolic' reading. Although we record both figures on our observation chart, it is only the systolic reading that generates a score.

These are some of the terms you may hear in relation to the blood pressure reading:

Normotension	Blood pressure within normal range
Hypotension	Blood pressure lower than normal range

Pulse

Age	Approximate range (beats per minute)
Newborn	120–160
1–12 Months	80–140
12 Months–2 years	80–130
2–6 years	75–120
6–12 years	75–110
Adolescent	60–100
Adult	60–100

Neurological assessment tool

A Alert
V Responds to voice or a change in the verbal response
P Responds to painful stimuli
U Unresponsive

Temperature

Low-grade pyrexia	Normal to 38°C
Moderate- to high-grade pyrexia	38–40°C
Hyperpyrexia	40°C and above

Appendix 4a An SBAR prompt sheet

S	**Situation** **I am calling about** (patient name and location) **The patient's resuscitation status is** (status) **The problem I am calling about is** ______________________________. I am afraid the patient is going to arrest. **I have just assessed the patient personally:** **Vital signs are**: Blood pressure _____/_____, Pulse ______, Respiration_____ and Temperature ______ **I am concerned about the:** Blood pressure because it is over 200 or less than 100 or 30 mmHg below usual. Pulse because it is over 140 or less than 50. Respiration because it is less than 5 or over 40. Temperature because it is less than 96 or over 104. Other:
B	**Background** **The patient's mental status is:** Alert and oriented to person place and time. Confused and cooperative or non-cooperative Agitated or combative Lethargic but conversant and able to swallow Stuporous and not talking clearly and possibly not able to swallow Comatose. Eyes closed. Not responding to stimulation. **The skin is:** Warm and dry Pale Mottled Clammy Extremities are cold Extremities are warm **The patient is not or is on oxygen.** The patient has been on ________ (l/min) or (%) oxygen for ______ minutes (hours). The oximeter is reading _______%. The oximeter does not detect a good pulse and is giving erratic readings.
A	**Assessment** **This is what I think the problem is: (** say what you think is the problem). **The problem seems to be cardiac infection neurologic respiratory _____.** **I am not sure what the problem is but the patient is deteriorating.** **The patient seems to be unstable and ma y get worse, we need to do something.**
R	**Recommendation** **I suggest or request that you** (say what you would like to see done). transfer the patient to critical care come to see the patient at this time. talk to the patient or family about resuscitation status. Other: **Are any tests needed:** Do you need any tests like CXR, ABG, ECG Others? **If a change in treatment is ordered then ask:** How often do you want vital signs? How long to you expect this problem will last? If the patient does not get better when would you want us to call again?

Confidential information, to be filed in patient's notes.

Appendix 4b The SBAR communication tool in poster format

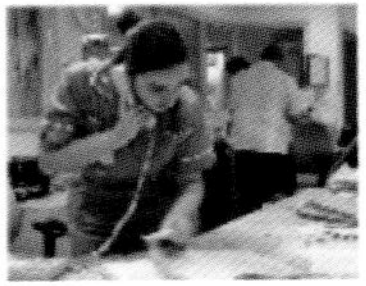

North Bristol NHS Trust NHS

SBAR Communication Tool

Situation Background Assessment Recommendation

Use the SBAR tool when making a referral to ensure good interprofessional communication

Situation
- Your details
- Patient details
- Location
- Reason for referral / admission

Background
- Admission diagnosis
- Relevant medical history
- Brief summary to date

Assessment (A–E)
Assess the patient : have a good look!

Airway - patent
Breathing - rate, cyanosis, % oxygen. Saturation, recent ABG results
Circulation - HR, BP, temp, IVI, urine output, Fluid balance
Disability - AVPU/cognition, BM, pain control, nutrition, continence, mobility
Exposure - wounds, drains, rash, swelling, pressure ulcers, infection control.

Recommendations
- State what you feel is needed
- Agree realistic time scale (urgent/ non urgent)

Have documents to hand

(you will inevitably be asked questions)

- Nursing notes
- Patient's clinical notes
- EWS Chart
- Fluid Chart
- Resuscitation status
- Treatment Plan / limitations

Have you considered:

- Repeat EWS
- Oxygen
- Patient position
- Fluid Chart
- Blood tests
- Frequency of obs
- ECG
- Blood glucose
- IV access

Don't forget to document the call –

Include : date, time, who you spoke to, bleep number and short summary of what was discussed.

Clear Communication
Safer Patients

Source: North Bristol NHS Trust and University Hospitals Bristol NHS Foundation Trust. Reproduced with permission.

Chapter 11

DOCUMENTATION

Communication Skills for Nurses, First Edition. Claire Boyd and Janet Dare
© 2014 John Wiley & Sons, Ltd. Published 2014 by John Wiley & Sons Ltd.

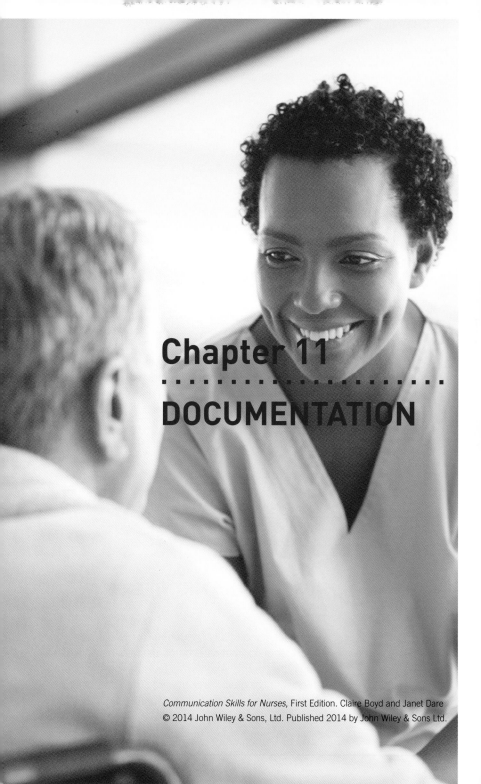

LEARNING OUTCOMES

By the end of this chapter you will have an understanding of the best practice in nursing documentation, record keeping and written communication.

Effective record-keeping is essential to facilitate robust communication between healthcare professionals. For example, a nurse writes on the care plan that the patient has undergone a full bed bath and that pressure areas are intact. There is no need for another nurse to complete this task.

Record-keeping may also provide evidence of care for incident investigations and legal cases. Comprehensive and clear records may not improve care, but if information regarding a patient's care has not been communicated then that care may indeed be compromised. For example, if the patient is unable to talk, how do we know that they have had a bed bath? Have the pressure areas been assessed?

The Nursing and Midwifery Council (2009) informs us that:

> Good record-keeping is an integral part of nursing and midwifery practice and is essential to the provision of safe and effective care.

NURSING AND MIDWIFERY COUNCIL

The Nursing and Midwifery Council (or NMC) is the UK regulator that safeguards the health and well-being of the public, and strives towards the consistent delivery of high-quality health care. The NMC's vision, mission and values also include nursing and midwifery students.

The NMC (2009) has also issued guidance for the principles of good record-keeping, stating that:

1. Handwriting should be legible.
2. All entries to records should be signed. In the case of written records, the person's name and job title should be printed alongside the first entry.
3. In line with local policy, you should put the date and time on all records. This should be in real time and chronological order and be as close to the actual time as possible.
4. Your records should be accurate and recorded in such a way that the meaning is clear.
5. Records should be factual and not include unnecessary abbreviations, jargon, meaningless phrases or irrelevant speculation.
6. You should use your professional judgement to decide what is relevant and what should be recorded.
7. You should record details of any assessments and reviews undertaken and provide clear evidence of the arrangements you have made for future and ongoing care. This should also include details of information given about care and treatment.
8. Records should identify any risks or problems that have arisen and show the action taken to deal with them.
9. You have a duty to communicate fully and effectively with your colleagues, ensuring that they have all the information they need about the people in your care.
10. You must not alter or destroy any records without being authorised to do so.
11. In the unlikely event that you need to alter your own or another healthcare professional's records, you must give your name and job title, and sign and date the original documentation. You should make sure that the alterations you make, and the original record, are clear and auditable.
12. Where appropriate, the person in your care, or their carer, should be involved in the record-keeping process.
13. The language that you use should be easily understood by the people in your care.

14 Records should be readable when photocopied or scanned.

15 You should not use coded expressions of sarcasm or humorous abbreviations to describe the people in your care.

16 You should not falsify records.

LEGAL ISSUES

Clinical records are part of the ongoing process of providing the correct patient care, but are frequently seen by nurses as a means of providing evidence for use in litigation cases, and are written in this style. Therefore they can be viewed in a negative and defensive way, rather than as part of the communication and care process.

It is true that nurses should always be able to give the rationale for the care they have provided, giving the intended goals for the interventions they have utilised, and reassessments where necessary. This is all as part of the nursing process. All care given must be recorded, as it has been suggested that 'if it wasn't documented, then it wasn't done' (Gasper, 2011).

During litigation cases, nurses may have to attend court to give evidence. Charges of negligence that cause patient harm are mostly heard in **civil courts**, whereas charges relating to intentionally harming a patient are heard in the **criminal courts**.

ROOT CAUSE ANALYSIS

When mistakes occur in the clinical setting, the clinical records are viewed as part of the investigation. This investigation is referred to as a **root cause analysis** whereby the incident is investigated in full, looking at what happened and when, what actions were taken and why they were taken. It also covers who was involved and who was informed about the incident. From this, solutions can be established and lessons learned; in essence, holes can be plugged. It has been found that, for the majority of incidents, a series of events and a wide range of contributory factors are involved, rather than the incident having one single cause.

ACCOUNTABILITY

At the end of your training, you will start to have interviews. One of the common questions asked during this process is: 'As a Registered Nurse, to whom are you accountable?' According to the NMC (2008), registered nurses are accountable to:

- the NMC to demonstrate fitness to practice and adherence to the code of conduct;
- their employer or trust to demonstrate fulfilment of their contractual agreement and that they are performing at the right standard for their role;
- the courts if there are claims of negligence or criminal acts (law);
- the patient and family.

NURSING DOCUMENTATION

Within the healthcare profession, whether you work in a hospital, care home or community setting, you will see many different charts, forms and types of documentation. Some of the most common documents you will come across during your training are the patient's hospital admission form (Appendix 1, Chapter 9), nursing care plans (such as the catheterisation care plan; see Appendix 5 at the end of this chapter), nursing activity forms (such as intentional rounding; see Appendix 6 at the end of this chapter), checklists (such as the observation chart; see Chapter 10), fluid balance chart and prescription (or drug) chart, to name just a few.

Another common document you may see in the hospital setting is the one required when preparing patients for discharge, known as discharge planning documentation. Ask to see this form while you are undertaking your hospital clinical placement.

Other documents you may come across are risk assessment documentation, such as:

- falls risk assessment (Appendix 7),
- bedrail risk assessment (Appendix 8),
- daily pressure ulcer risk assessment (Appendix 9),
- VTE risk assessment (Appendix 10).

All the above appendices can be found at the end of this chapter.

GLOSSARY

VTE
Venous thrombotic embolism.

Look at these appendices at the end of this chapter. It is good to get to grips with the many documents you will come across. You will notice that the VTE risk assessment (Appendix 10) gives instructions for recording the information electronically. In today's healthcare system, drives are being made to implement paperless records. Whether electronic or written on paper, the principles of record-keeping remain the same. As a student, you will be shown how to complete this paperwork with your assessor. This is because, even if you are unable to sign any of these documents, you can start to build a working knowledge of them.

TEST YOUR KNOWLEDGE

1. List six of the 16 NMC principles of good record-keeping.
2. If a formal investigation is undertaken, what is it called?
3. Charges of negligence that cause patient harm are mostly heard in ____?
4. Charges relating to intentionally harming a patient are heard in the ____?
5. As a registered nurse, to whom are you accountable?
6. What do the abbreviations VTE mean?

KEY POINTS

- Record-keeping
- NMC principles of good record-keeping
- Legal issues
- Accountability
- Nursing documentation

Bibliography

Glasper, A. (2011) Improving record-keeping: important lessons for nurses. *British Journal of Nursing* 20(14), 886–887.

National Patient Safety Agency (2011) *Patient Safety First 2008–2010. The Campaign Review.* NPSA, London.

Nursing and Midwifery Council (2008) *The Code: Standards of Conduct, Performance and Ethics for Nurses and Midwives.* NMC, London; www.nmc-uk.org/code.

Nursing and Midwifery Council (2009) *Record Keeping: Guidance for Nurses and Midwives.* NMC, London.

Reason, J. (2000) Human error: models and management. *British Medical Journal* 320(7237), 768–770.

Vincent, C. (2010) *Patient Safety*, 2nd edn. Wiley Blackwell, Oxford.

Appendix 5 Catheterisation care plan documentation

Addressograph:

Urinary Catheter Care Plan

North Bristol **NHS**
NHS Trust

Ward: Date:

Indication for catheter (look for the indication on catheter insertion sticker)
- ☐ Accurate fluid balance (critically ill?)
- ☐ Urine retention
- ☐ Urinary tract haemorrhage
- ☐ Major Surgery
- ☐ Palliative
- ☐ Skin breakdown from incontinence
- ☐ Other (please specify):

Date of insertion: ....

Estimated date for removal or change: ....

	Date																					
	Action	E	L	N	E	L	N	E	L	N	E	L	N	E	L	N	E	L	N	E	L	N
1.	**Hand hygiene** Before and after each patient contact **(document every shift)**																					
2.	**Catheter hygiene** Clean catheter site **at least once a day** as per policy CP1f																					
3.	**Drainage bag position** Check position above floor but below bladder level to prevent reflux or contamination and assist drainage **(every shift)**																					
4.	**Sampling (needle-free) aseptically via catheter port (document whenever sample is obtained)**																					
5.	**Manipulation -Securing the catheter** Check catheter secured using a fixation device using aseptic technique and comfortable for patient. Leg straps must be removed at night**(document every shift)**																					
6.	**Manipulation - Catheter drainage bag emptying** Empty at least **twice daily (document twice daily minimum)** Gloves and apron must be worn Clean container used every time Decontaminate port before emptying Avoid touching drainage tap Decontaminate hands after taking gloves and apron off																					
7.	**Manipulation - Changing drainage bag** Urine drainage bags and valves must be dated and changed at least **every 7 days (document weekly minimum)**																					
8.	**Catheter needed?** Review **daily**, remove as soon as possible **(document daily)**																					
	Please initial after each action																					

Record actions each shift, daily or weekly as indicated on the checklist above. Record ✓=yes **✗**=no in the boxes.
Initial after each review at the bottom of the care plan.

SESv3. 15.02.11

lgd

Date	Variance	Sign

Guidance

Hand hygiene 5 moments
Before touching patient
Before clean/ aseptic procedures
After body fluid exposure
After touching patient
After touching patient surroundings

Sampling
Perform aseptically via the needle-free catheter port.
Catheter manipulation (any action which involves touching the catheter system)
Examination gloves must be worn to manipulate a catheter, and manipulation should be preceded and followed by hand decontamination.
Maintain a closed system
Connection between catheter and drainage bag must not be broken except for good clinical reason e.g. changing drainage bag.
Single use non-drainable night bag may be used at night.
Recording
Record urinary output on fluid chart if appropriate.
Encourage good fluid intake.
Report poor output, (adequate output is 0.5 ml per kg of patient's body weight per hour e.g.33 mls if patient weighs 66 kg).
Report any changes in colour e.g. blood.
Self management of hygiene & emptying
Following education and help if appropriate.
After removal of catheter
Ensure patient is within easy reach of a toilet or voiding receptacle.
Monitor intake and output, ensure patient is comfortable and feels that the bladder is empty after voiding.
Record episodes of incontinence.

For further information refer to: Policy for Adult Urethral Catheterisation and Supra-pubic Re-catheterisation Policy CP 1f

SESv3. 15.02.11

Source: North Bristol NHS Trust and University Hospitals Bristol NHS Foundation Trust. Reproduced with permission.

Appendix 6 Intentional rounding checklist tool for falls

8/7/2011

North Bristol NHS
NHS Trust

Intentional Rounding Checklist Tool for Falls

Name	
Hospital Number	Falls leaflet given ☐ Continence checked ☐ Supervision for toileting documented in notes ☐
DOB	Doctors asked to review medication ☐ Referral made to physiotherapy ☐ Vision checked ☐
Ward	**Round every 1 hr for High risk** **2 hr for Medium risk** (Circle times below and initial after each round)

Date: Time:	8 am	9 am	10 am	11 am	12 n	1 pm	2 pm	3 pm	4 pm	5 pm	6 pm	7 pm	8 pm	9 pm	10 pm	11 pm	12 mn	1 am	2 am	3 am	4 am	5 am	6 am	7 am
ARE YOU COMFORTABLE? Re-positioned 2 hourly																								
DO YOU NEED THE TOILET?																								
DO YOU HAVE ANY PAIN?																								
Orientated= O (please indicate) confused =C asleep=A																								
WOULD YOU LIKE A DRINK? Fluids offered																								
Call bell within reach **IF YOU NEED ME, PLEASE PRESS THIS BUTTON.**																								
Bed rails down/bed lowest position																								
Footwear checked																								
IS THERE ANYTHING ELSE I CAN DO? I HAVE THE TIME																								

Date: Time:	8 am	9 am	10 am	11 am	12 n	1 pm	2 pm	3 pm	4 pm	5 pm	6 pm	7 pm	8 pm	9 pm	10 pm	11 pm	12 mn	1 am	2 am	3 am	4 am	5 am	6 am	7 am
ARE YOU COMFORTABLE? Re-positioned 2 hourly																								
DO YOU NEED THE TOILET?																								
DO YOU HAVE ANY PAIN?																								
Orientated= O (please indicate) confused =C asleep=A																								
WOULD YOU LIKE A DRINK? Fluids offered																								
Call bell within reach **IF YOU NEED ME, PLEASE PRESS THIS BUTTON.**																								
Bed rails down/bed lowest position																								
Footwear checked																								
IS THERE ANYTHING ELSE I CAN DO? I HAVE THE TIME																								

Date: Time:	8 am	9 am	10 am	11 am	12 n	1 pm	2 pm	3 pm	4 pm	5 pm	6 pm	7 pm	8 pm	9 pm	10 pm	11 pm	12 mn	1 am	2 am	3 am	4 am	5 am	6 am	7 am
ARE YOU COMFORTABLE? Re-positioned 2 hourly																								
DO YOU NEED THE TOILET?																								
DO YOU HAVE ANY PAIN?																								
Orientated= O (please indicate) confused =C asleep=A																								
WOULD YOU LIKE A DRINK? Fluids offered																								
Call bell within reach **IF YOU NEED ME, PLEASE PRESS THIS BUTTON.**																								
Bed rails down/bed lowest position																								
Footwear checked																								
IS THERE ANYTHING ELSE I CAN DO? I HAVE THE TIME																								

Date: Time:	8 am	9 am	10 am	11 am	12 n	1 pm	2 pm	3 pm	4 pm	5 pm	6 pm	7 pm	8 pm	9 pm	10 pm	11 pm	12 mn	1 am	2 am	3 am	4 am	5 am	6 am	7 am
ARE YOU COMFORTABLE? Re-positioned 2 hourly																								
DO YOU NEED THE TOILET?																								
DO YOU HAVE ANY PAIN?																								
Orientated= O (please indicate) confused =C asleep=A																								
WOULD YOU LIKE A DRINK? Fluids offered																								
Call bell within reach **IF YOU NEED ME, PLEASE PRESS THIS BUTTON.**																								
Bed rails down/bed lowest position																								
Footwear checked																								
IS THERE ANYTHING ELSE I CAN DO? I HAVE THE TIME																								

Comments:

Source: North Bristol NHS Trust and University Hospitals Bristol NHS Foundation Trust. Reproduced with permission.

Appendix 7 Falls risk assessment tool

North Bristol NHS
NHS Trust

Falls Risk Assessment Tool

Patient Name:	Hospital no:	Ward:	Date:

Addressograph:

- **Patient risk assessment must be completed on admission and weekly as a minimum.**
- **If patient's clinical condition changes or changes ward, please reassess.**
- **Give NBT Patient Falls Prevention leaflet to all patients**

Risk Factors
Please tick if any of the risk factors are present below:

HIGH RISK						
	Date					
	Acute confusion/delirium					
	Fall in hospital this admission					
	Attempting to stand or walk unaided when not safe to do so					
	Using your clinical judgment, the patient would benefit from intentional rounding					

If **any** factors present → Intentional Rounding Minimum **HOURLY**

MEDIUM RISK						
	Fall as the presenting complaint for admission					
	Chronic confusion or dementia					
	Unsteady when walking/turning					
	Prescribed sedative medication					
	Under influence or withdrawing from alcohol/drugs					
	The multi-disciplinary team feels the patient is at risk of falling					

If **3 factors or above** present, and **none** higher → Complete **Intentional Rounding** Minimum **2 HOURLY**

If **less than 3** factors present → Complete **Falls Care** Plan **EVERY SHIFT**

LOWER						
	Previous falls (not related to presentation or admission					
	Any other concerns (previous fracture, post-operative)					
	Relatives anxious about falls					

If **any** factors present, and **none** higher → Complete **Falls Care** Plan **EVERY SHIFT**

Minimal RISK						
	None of the above risk factors present					

Re-assess **weekly** or if **change** in clinical **condition**

Weekly record of risk assessment:

Date	Time	Risk level (tick)				Staff name		Designation (tick)			
		Minimal risk	Lower	Medium	High	Signature	PRINT NAME	HCA*	Student nurse*	AP*	RGN

* must be countersigned

SES.v10.6/06/2011

13/12/2010

RVJ0804 lgd

Source: North Bristol NHS Trust and University Hospitals Bristol NHS Foundation Trust. Reproduced with permission.

Appendix 8 Adult patient bedrail risk assessment

North Bristol NHS
NHS Trust

ADULT PATIENT BEDRAIL RISK ASSESSMENT		
Directorate		Patient Details *(Affix label if available)*
Ward		

The Falls Risk Assessment must be completed prior to completion of this bedrail assessment.

Staff should use the bedrail risk assessment in addition to their **professional judgement** to consider the risks and benefits for Individual patients.

RISK FACTOR Please record answers to these questions in box ✓=yes x=no	**USE OF BEDRAILS**	**NOTES**	**Date** / **Initial of Reviewer**					
Patient is independently mobile	**Bedrails not to be used**	Check patient has not requested use of bedrails						
Patient **is likely to** attempt to get out of bed alone	**Bedrails not to be used**	Use height adjustable bed to suit patients requirements						
Patient has previously attempted to climb over bedrails	**Bedrails not to be used**	Consider use of low height bed						
Patient has uncontrolled limb movements / restless/ significantly confused	**Bedrails not to be used**	Consider use of low height bed						
Patient has difficulty rolling over in bed	**Bedrails not to be used**							
Patient **is not likely** to attempt to get out of bed alone	**Consider use of Bedrails**	Optional use of protective bedrail bumpers						
Patient has disruption to their spatial or visual awareness	**Consider use of Bedrails**	Optional use of protective bedrail bumpers						
Patient has a fear of falling out of bed whilst asleep	**Consider use of Bedrails**	Ensure bedrails are securely fitted in matching pairs, and in good working order						
Patient is recovering from an anaesthetic	**Bedrails to be used**	Ensure bedrails are securely fitted in matching pairs, and in good working order						
Patient has requested bedrails or uses bedrails at home	**Bedrails to be used**	Ensure bedrails are securely fitted in matching pairs, and in good working order						
Patient is unconscious or completely immobile	**Bedrails to be used**	Ensure bedrails are securely fitted in matching pairs, and in good working order						
	Please put bed rail sign above the bed	**BED RAILS USED (tick and initial)**						
		BED RAILS NOT USED (tick and initial)						

If risk factors conflict e.g. Patient is independently mobile and the patient has requested bedrails, or uses bedrails at home, staff need to use their **professional judgement** to consider the risks and benefits for individual patients and document.

Consideration should be given to other control measures when completing this assessment.

Report any faulty bed rails to the Huntleigh Equipment Library for repair as soon as possible

Source: North Bristol NHS Trust and University Hospitals Bristol NHS Foundation Trust. Reproduced with permission.

Appendix 9 Daily pressure ulcer risk assessment tool

Daily Pressure Ulcer Risk Assessment Tool

North Bristol NHS
NHS Trust

Small Addressograph:

Patient surname:

First name:

Hospital no.:

Ward: **Date:**

Transferred to ward: **Transfer date:**

- **Risk assessment must be completed within 6 hours of admission**
- **Must be re-assessed daily as a minimum.**
- **Re-assess if clinical condition changes / transferred to other wards**

Daily risk factors (NICE guidance CG29 2005)

Please tick (✓) each day if risk factors are present and complete the daily record of risk assessment below:

Risk	Risk factor	Date	Date	Date	Date		SKIN check frequency	Recommended equipment & therapy
High Risk	Existing pressure ulcer or previous history of pressure ulcers					**If any factors present**	**SKIN check 2 HOURLY Minimum** Discuss pressure ulcer prevention with patient/ relative - MDT consideration	Electric profiling bed frame with dynamic replacement mattress. Dynamic mattress may vary: Autologic, Nimbus 2 or Nimbus 3. Repose – add foot protectors (if necessary)
	Reduced responsiveness to verbal or painful stimulus							
	Pain – that reduces mobility							
	Epidural							
	Skin moist nearly all of the time (e.g. skin moist despite containment interventions for incontinence)							
	Confined to bed or chair most of the time							
	Makes only occasional or no change in position without assistance							
	Eating less than 1/2 of meals							
	Needs moderate to maximum assistance in moving with high risk of friction against surface							
	Clinical obesity - BMI >40							
Medium Risk	Sensory impairment					***If any factors present and none higher***	**SKIN check 4 HOURLY Minimum** Discuss pressure ulcer prevention with patient/ relative - MDT consideration.	Electric profiling bed frame and pressure reducing static mattress. Repose – add foot protectors (if necessary) Encourage mobility. Ensure seating assessed to reflect patient needs. Regular skin checks required.
	Skin often moist (e.g. incontinent but containment interventions satisfactory)							
	Walks occasionally							
	Mobility limited							
	Generally eats only half of any meal							
	Needs some assistance to move with some contact against surface							
	Vascular disease							
	Severe chronic or palliative illness							
Low Risk	Steroids					***If any factors present and none higher***	**SKIN check DAILY Minimum** Discuss skin care with patient/ relative - MDT consideration	Static bed frame and pressure reducing static mattress e.g. softform / pentaflex.
	No sensory deficit to pain							
	Skin rarely moist							
	Walks frequently							
	No limitation in mobility							
	Moves in bed & chair independently – able to lift self over surface with low friction risk							
	Eats most of every meal							

Registered nursing staff must use their own clinical judgement to step down from dynamic mattresses if it is compromising patient rehabilitation. These recommendations are guidance only. Deviation from care must be recorded on page 4.

Daily record of risk assessment

Date:	Time:	Risk level (tick):			Staff name:		Designation (tick): ** must be countersigned*				
		Low	Medium	High	Signature:	PRINT NAME:	HCA*	AP*	RGN / RGM	AHP	Student Nurse*

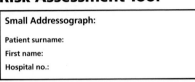

SKIN bundle for pressure ulcer prevention

Every box must be completed with a Y / N or a sample code given on the form. If you are unable to complete **ANY** of the boxes due to the patient being off the ward, please use the exception code Off Ward (OW).

E Early	**L** Left side bed	**R** Right side bed	**SR** Semi-recumbent	**LR** Log Roll	**U** Unable due to physical condition (please document details in clinical record)
L Late	**B** Back	**SIB** Sat in bed	**SU** Stood up	**F** Front	
N Night	**RF** Refused	**SIC** Sit in chair	**I** Independent		

Date:													
SKIN check: circle the relevant frequency		**Daily / 4 hourly / 2 hourly**			**Daily / 4 hourly / 2 hourly**			**Daily / 4 hourly / 2 hourly**			**Daily / 4 hourly / 2 hourly**		
Time:		E	L	N	E	L	N	E	L	N	E	L	N
Surface	Electric profiling bed frame in use (Y / N)												
	Mattress (S = Static, N2, N3, AL)												
	Dynamic mattress pump working (Y / N / NA)												
	Cushion (F = Foam, R = Roho, A = Aura, NA)												
	Do you have recommended equipment e.g. bed frame, dynamic mattress or cushion (Y / N)												
	Sheets (wrinkle free, clean). Do not tuck in / no fitted sheets on dynamic mattresses (Y/ N)												
Keep moving	Skin assessed: Visual check (min daily low risk, 4 hours medium risk, 1-2 hourly high risk) (Y / N)												
	Remove anti-embolic stockings to inspect heels												
	Position changed - use codes above (min daily low risk, 4 hours medium risk, 1-2 hourly high risk)												
Incontinence	Clean and dry: Visual check minimum 4 hours (Y / N)												
	Catheter system checked (Y / N / NA)												
	Regular toileting offered (Y / N / NA)												
	Episode of faecal incontinence (Y / N / NA)												
Nutrition	Malnutrition Screening Tool completed within the last week (Y / N). If *No*, complete the tool.												
	Nutritional supplements offered (Y / N / NA)												
	Received no nutrition > 3 days (Y / N) If *Yes*, consider artificial nutrition.												
	Completed by: (Please initial)												

(continued)

Appendix 9 *(Continued)*

Prevention of Deterioration

This form is to monitor pressure ulcers on a daily basis

Note: Record Grade/Category 1 pressure ulcer on date when identified in appropriate table below and amend the ward Safety Cross. If a higher grade/category is identified/or a grade/category 1 deteriorates to grade/category 2, 3 or 4, please generate a new eAIMS form and commence a Wound Assessment and Management Care Plan.

On deterioration to grade/category 3 or 4 please refer to Tissue Viability team via ICE.

Do not reverse the grade/category; from a higher grade/category to a lower grade/category.

Grade/category 1:

Intact skin with non-blanchable erythema. Darkly pigmented skin may not have visible blanching; it's colour may differ from surrounding area.

EPUAP2009

Record how many grade/category 1 pressure ulcers on each day. Two members of staff should assess and agree any new areas of skin changes. **Tick (✓) if completed and cross (x) if not completed.** NICE Guidance 2005 Essence of Care 2010	*Use the correct Date column for day: Column 1 for Day 1 etc.*			
	Date	Date	Date	Date
Share information with colleagues; include in handover/safety briefing				
Remove pressure from affected area(s)				
Remove friction/shearing				
Remove moisture				
Generate eAIMS form when pressure ulcer is identified				
Initials:				

Body Map

Please mark the body map daily with an X to indicate the position of the pressure ulcer with a number to the side to indicate the grade/category of the pressure ulcer present in that position, as shown below.

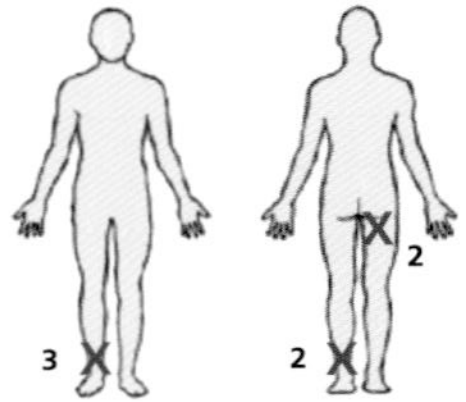

Date:
Complete once daily

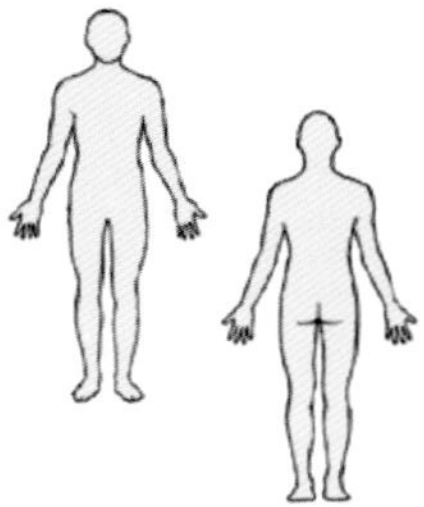

☐ No new pink / No new darker skin

☐ Remove anti-embolic stockings daily to inspect heels

Date:
Complete once daily

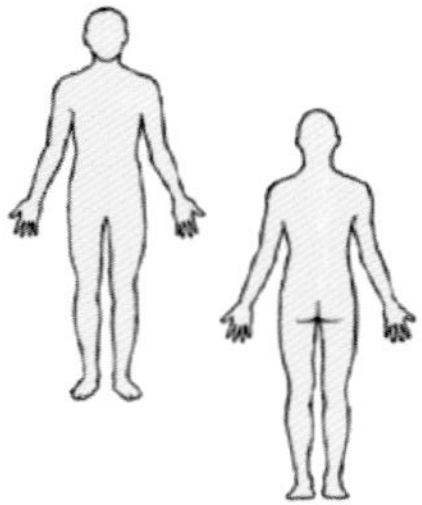

☐ No new pink / No new darker skin

☐ Remove anti-embolic stockings daily to inspect heels

Date:
Complete once daily

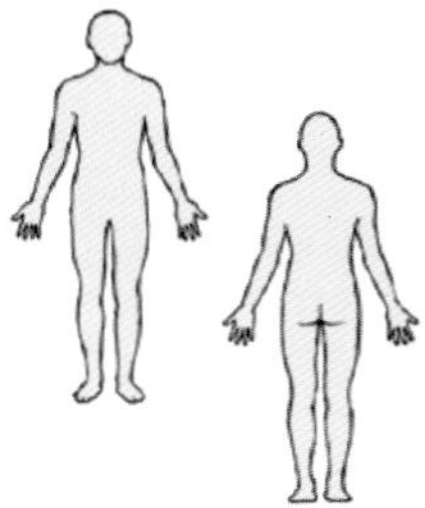

☐ No new pink / No new darker skin

☐ Remove anti-embolic stockings daily to inspect heels

Date:
Complete once daily

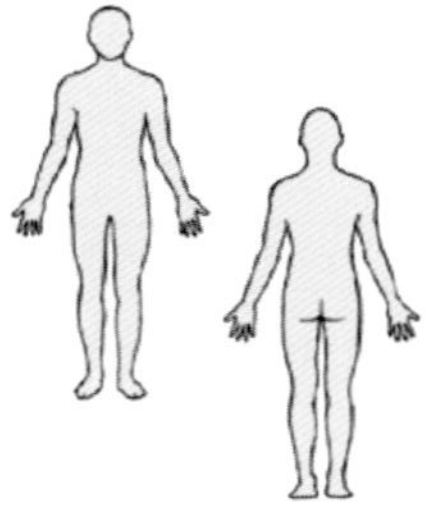

☐ No new pink / No new darker skin

☐ Remove anti-embolic stockings daily to inspect heels

Deviation from Clinical Record

Date	Comments	Signature	Printed Name	Designation

References:

European Pressure Ulcer Advisory Panel and National Pressure Ulcer Advisory Panel
International Guideline Prevention of Pressure Ulcers. Quick Reference Guide (2009)

Department of Health
Essence of Care: Benchmarks for prevention and management of Presure Ulcers (2010)

Institute for Innovation and Improvement High Impact Actions for Nursing and Midwifery
Your Skin Matters (2010)

National Institute for Health and Clinical Excellence (2005)
Clinical Guideline 29 developed by the Royal College of Nursing

National Institute for Health and Clinical Excellence (2005)
Quick Reference Guide. The Prevention and Treatment of Pressure Ulcers

Source: North Bristol NHS Trust and University Hospitals Bristol NHS Foundation Trust. Reproduced with permission.

Appendix 10 Revised VTE risk assessment audit guide

North Bristol NHS
NHS Trust

<u>Revised VTE Risk Assessment Audit Guide</u>

Initial screen requires all fields to be entered before proceeding by clicking 'NEXT'.

Date of audit has a calendar drop down.

Auditor Name is free text.

Auditor Job Title / Role has a drop-down list which includes 'Pharmacist'.

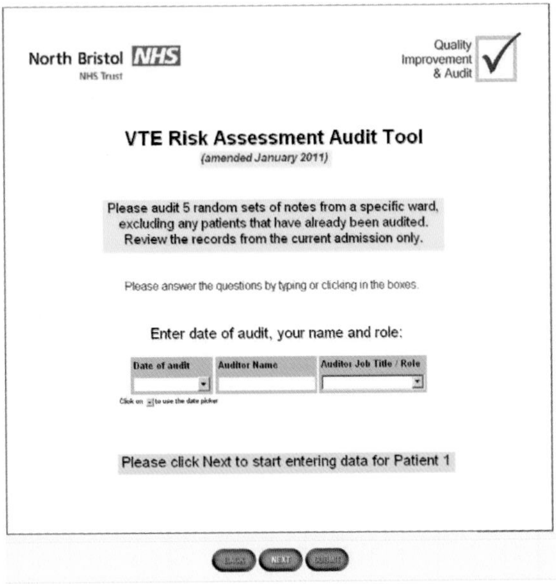
North Bristol NHS
NHS Trust

Quality
Improvement
& Audit

VTE Risk Assessment Audit Tool

(amended January 2011)

Please audit 5 random sets of notes from a specific ward, excluding any patients that have already been audited. Review the records from the current admission only.

Please answer the questions by typing or clicking in the boxes.

Enter date of audit, your name and role:

Date of audit	Auditor Name	Auditor Job Title / Role

Click on ▼ to use the date picker

Please click Next to start entering data for Patient 1

NEXT

Prepared by: Lloyd Mayers + Fiona Blain (pharmacy) 10 Jan 2011 and updated 16 Feb 2011
Authorised by: NBT Thrombosis Committee 12 Jan 2011
Review date: Jan 2013

North Bristol NHS
NHS Trust

Revised VTE Risk Assessment Audit Guide

Data entry for each patient contains a mixture of free text fields, drop-downs, dependent drop-downs and check boxes.

Enter patient number as free text, this should include the S, F or N prefix.

Enter DoB as free text, this must be in the dd/mm/yyyy format.

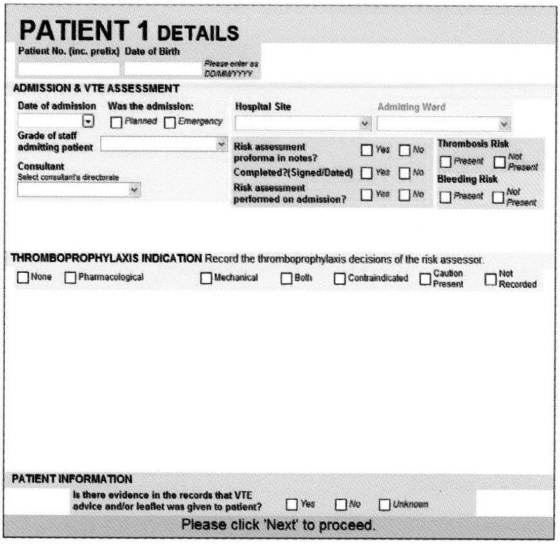

Select either Planned or Emergency admission check box.

Grade of staff admitting patient has a drop-down. Dr's are listed a F1, F2, Middle Grade and Consultant. Middle Grade are all Dr's not classed as F1, F2 or Consultant.

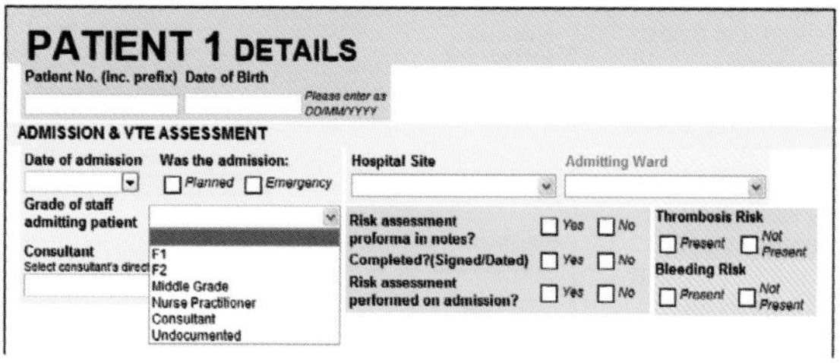

Date of admission has a calendar drop down.

Site of admitting ward has a drop down. The available admitting wards are dependent on the site selected.

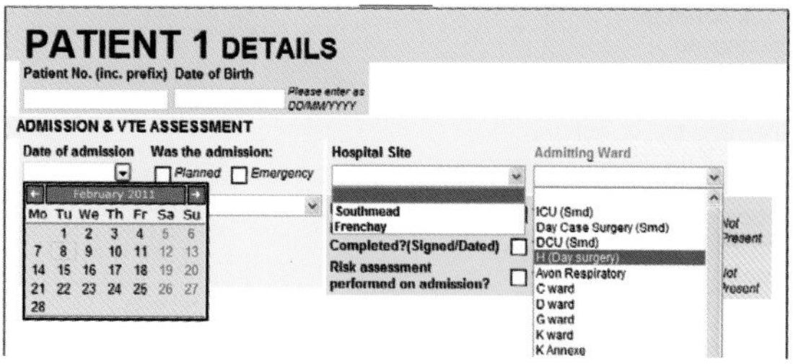

Prepared by: Lloyd Mayers + Fiona Blain (pharmacy) 10 Jan 2011 and updated 16 Feb 2011
Authorised by: NBT Thrombosis Committee 12 Jan 2011
Review date: Jan 2013

(continued)

Appendix 10 *(Continued)*

North Bristol NHS
NHS Trust

Revised VTE Risk Assessment Audit Guide

Consultant code is the 2 or 3 character IHS code.

Available Consultant codes are dependent on the directorate selected.

Status of risk assessment consists of three pairs of 'yes' or 'no' checkboxes.

The proforma must have a tick, be signed and dated to qualify as completed.
If 'no' is ticked for 'proforma in notes' then some subsequent fields will become unavailable.

If 'no' is entered at any stage then an orange action box appears. Complete this action (see introductory notes) and check 'confirmed' check box.

Check boxes for documented thrombosis and bleeding risk. As either 'present' or 'not present' if ***no ticks present in relevant section of proforma then select 'not present'.***

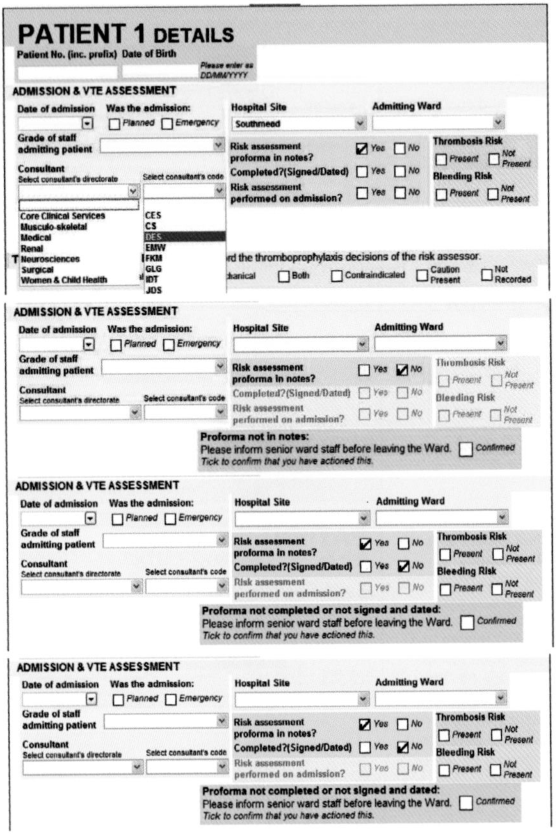

PATIENT 1 DETAILS
Patient No. (inc. prefix) Date of Birth
Please enter as DD/MM/YYYY
ADMISSION & VTE ASSESSMENT
Date of admission Was the admission: Planned Emergency
Hospital Site Southmead
Admitting Ward
Grade of staff admitting patient
Risk assessment proforma in notes? Yes No
Completed?(Signed/Dated) Yes No
Risk assessment performed on admission? Yes No
Thrombosis Risk Present Not Present
Bleeding Risk Present Not Present
Consultant
Select consultant's directorate
Select consultant's code
Core Clinical Services
Musculo-skeletal
Medical
Renal
Neurosciences
Surgical
Women & Child Health
CES
CS
DES
EMW
FKM
GLG
IDT
JDS
rd the thromboprophylaxis decisions of the risk assessor.
hanical Both Contraindicated Caution Present Not Recorded
Proforma not in notes:
Please inform senior ward staff before leaving the Ward. Confirmed
Tick to confirm that you have actioned this.
Proforma not completed or not signed and dated:
Please inform senior ward staff before leaving the Ward. Confirmed
Tick to confirm that you have actioned this.

Prepared by: Lloyd Mayers + Fiona Blain (pharmacy) 10 Jan 2011 and updated 16 Feb 2011
Authorised by: NBT Thrombosis Committee 12 Jan 2011
Review date: Jan 2013

North Bristol NHS
NHS Trust

Revised VTE Risk Assessment Audit Guide

If the risk assessment proforma is incomplete then the 'Not recorded' box in Thromboprophylaxis indicated box may be ticked.

Thromboprophylaxis indication consists of 'None', 'Pharmacological', 'Mechanical', 'Both', or 'Not Recorded' only one of these may be checked.

In addition 'Contraindicated' or 'Caution present' may be checked.

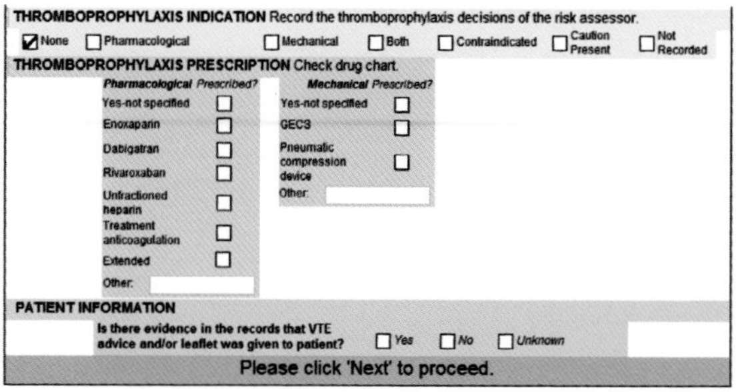

THROMBOPROPHYLAXIS INDICATION Record the thromboprophylaxis decisions of the risk assessor.

☑ None ☐ Pharmacological ☐ Mechanical ☐ Both ☐ Contraindicated ☐ Caution Present ☐ Not Recorded

THROMBOPROPHYLAXIS PRESCRIPTION Check drug chart.

Pharmacological Prescribed?: Yes-not specified ☐; Enoxaparin ☐; Dabigatran ☐; Rivaroxaban ☐; Unfractioned heparin ☐; Treatment anticoagulation ☐; Extended ☐; Other:

Mechanical Prescribed?: Yes-not specified ☐; GECS ☐; Pneumatic compression device ☐; Other:

PATIENT INFORMATION

Is there evidence in the records that VTE advice and/or leaflet was given to patient? ☐ Yes ☐ No ☐ Unknown

Please click 'Next' to proceed.

Enter the information documented on the risk assessment proforma.

Depending on the Thromboprophylaxis indicated, dependent check boxes will be available. Check boxes corresponding to prophylaxis decisions documented in the risk assessment proforma.

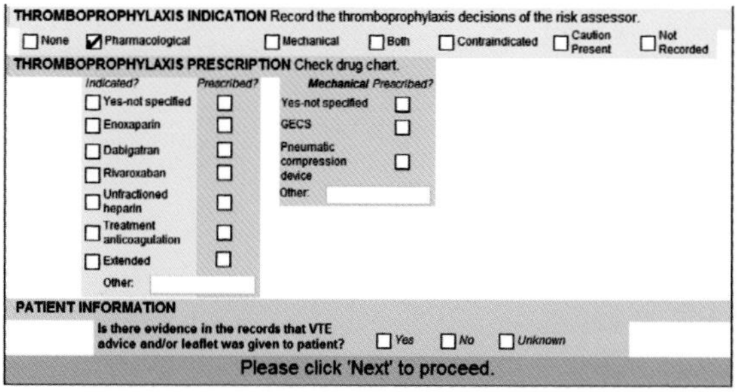

THROMBOPROPHYLAXIS INDICATION Record the thromboprophylaxis decisions of the risk assessor.

☐ None ☑ Pharmacological ☐ Mechanical ☐ Both ☐ Contraindicated ☐ Caution Present ☐ Not Recorded

THROMBOPROPHYLAXIS PRESCRIPTION Check drug chart.

Indicated? / Prescribed?: ☐ Yes-not specified ☐; ☐ Enoxaparin ☐; ☐ Dabigatran ☐; ☐ Rivaroxaban ☐; ☐ Unfractioned heparin ☐; ☐ Treatment anticoagulation ☐; ☐ Extended ☐; Other:

Mechanical Prescribed?: Yes-not specified ☐; GECS ☐; Pneumatic compression device ☐; Other:

PATIENT INFORMATION

Is there evidence in the records that VTE advice and/or leaflet was given to patient? ☐ Yes ☐ No ☐ Unknown

Please click 'Next' to proceed.

Prepared by: Lloyd Mayers + Fiona Blain (pharmacy) 10 Jan 2011 and updated 16 Feb 2011
Authorised by: NBT Thrombosis Committee 12 Jan 2011
Review date: Jan 2013

(continued)

Appendix 10 *(Continued)*

North Bristol NHS
NHS Trust

Revised VTE Risk Assessment Audit Guide

Where prophylaxis is documented as required but the agent is not specified select 'Yes-not specified'.

Check boxes for prescribed pharmacological and mechanical prophylaxis are available independently of documented indication. Check boxes corresponding to prescribed items.

Where patients are prescribed treatment anticoagulation with fondaparinux, warfarin, treatment dose enoxaparin, iv heparin, etc select 'Treatment anticoagulation'. If 'bleeding risk' (or similar) has been ticked by person completing proforma count this as contraindication (and put treatment anticoagulation in comment box). If treatment anticoagulation prescribed but 'bleeding risk' not ticked then leave contraindication blank.

Only select 'extended' as prescribed if this is indicated on the chart, i.e. for .... days.

THROMBOPROPHYLAXIS INDICATION Record the thromboprophylaxis decisions of the risk assessor.

☐ None ☐ Pharmacological ☑ Mechanical ☐ Both ☐ Contraindicated ☐ Caution Present ☐ Not Recorded

THROMBOPROPHYLAXIS PRESCRIPTION Check drug chart.

Pharmacological	*Prescribed?*	*Indicated?*	*Prescribed?*
Yes-not specified	☐	☐ Yes-not specified	☐
Enoxaparin	☐	☐ GECS	☐
Dabigatran	☐	☐ Pneumatic compression device	☐
Rivaroxaban	☐	Other:	
Unfractioned heparin	☐		
Treatment anticoagulation	☐		
Extended	☐		
Other:			

PATIENT INFORMATION

Is there evidence in the records that VTE advice and/or leaflet was given to patient? ☐ Yes ☐ No ☐ Unknown

Please click 'Next' to proceed.

THROMBOPROPHYLAXIS INDICATION Record the thromboprophylaxis decisions of the risk assessor.

☐ None ☐ Pharmacological ☐ Mechanical ☑ Both ☐ Contraindicated ☐ Caution Present ☐ Not Recorded

THROMBOPROPHYLAXIS PRESCRIPTION Check drug chart.

Indicated?	*Prescribed?*	*Indicated?*	*Prescribed?*
☐ Yes-not specified	☐	☐ Yes-not specified	☐
☐ Enoxaparin	☐	☐ GECS	☐
☐ Dabigatran	☐	☐ Pneumatic compression device	☐
☐ Rivaroxaban	☐	Other:	
☐ Unfractioned heparin	☐		
☐ Treatment anticoagulation	☐		
☐ Extended	☐		
Other:			

PATIENT INFORMATION

Is there evidence in the records that VTE advice and/or leaflet was given to patient? ☐ Yes ☐ No ☐ Unknown

Please click 'Next' to proceed.

Prepared by: Lloyd Mayers + Fiona Blain (pharmacy) 10 Jan 2011 and updated 16 Feb 2011
Authorised by: NBT Thrombosis Committee 12 Jan 2011
Review date: Jan 2013

North Bristol NHS
NHS Trust

Revised VTE Risk Assessment Audit Guide

When either 'contraindication' or 'caution present' is selected a free text box will be available.

Concisely document the reason for this decision in the available box. Where a reason is not documented in the risk assessment proforma then leave blank.

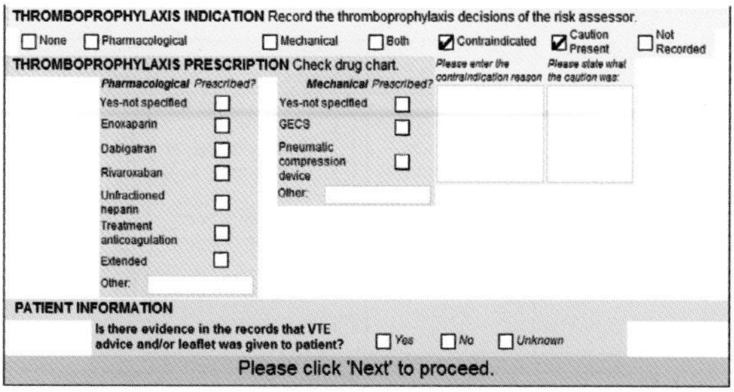
THROMBOPROPHYLAXIS INDICATION Record the thromboprophylaxis decisions of the risk assessor.

☐ None ☐ Pharmacological ☐ Mechanical ☐ Both ☑ Contraindicated ☑ Caution Present ☐ Not Recorded

THROMBOPROPHYLAXIS PRESCRIPTION Check drug chart.

Pharmacological Prescribed?		Mechanical Prescribed?		Please enter the contraindication reason	Please state what the caution was:
Yes-not specified	☐	Yes-not specified	☐		
Enoxaparin	☐	GECS	☐		
Dabigatran	☐	Pneumatic compression device	☐		
Rivaroxaban	☐	Other:			
Unfractioned heparin	☐				
Treatment anticoagulation	☐				
Extended	☐				
Other:					

PATIENT INFORMATION

Is there evidence in the records that VTE advice and/or leaflet was given to patient? ☐ Yes ☐ No ☐ Unknown

Please click 'Next' to proceed.

- Tick unknown for patient information leaflet unless documented in the notes as being given e.g. if preparing for surgery leaflet has been ticked on pre-admission paperwork.

- If surgical directorate is selected an additional field for 'post operative VTE risk assessment' will be available (under the Consultant directorate and IHS code drop downs). Yes, No or N/A can be selected. Check if the patient is post operative (a 'operation note' proforma should be in the notes if this is the case, example on right).

  1. If this is not present select N/A

  If the proforma is present check that the D.V.T prophylaxis been completed ***either as Yes ☑ or No ☑***

  2. If either has been ticked select Yes in this section of the audit
  3. If neither has been ticked select No in this section of the audit.

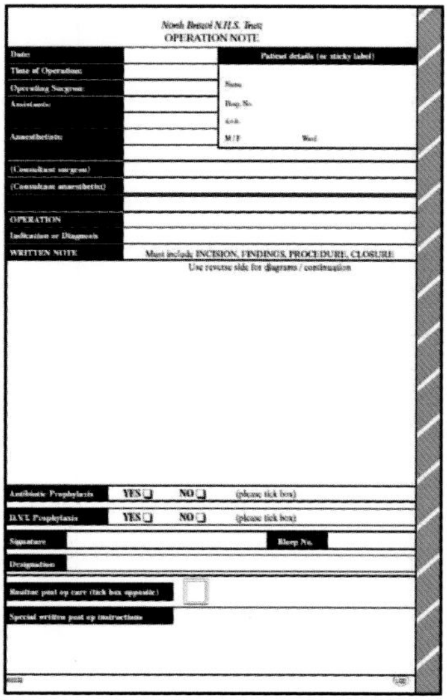
North Bristol N.H.S. Trust
OPERATION NOTE

Date: | Patient details (or sticky label)
Time of Operation:
Operating Surgeon:
Assistants:
Anaesthetists:
(Consultant surgeon)
(Consultant anaesthetist)
OPERATION
Indication or Diagnosis
WRITTEN NOTE — Must include INCISION, FINDINGS, PROCEDURE, CLOSURE
Use reverse side for diagrams / continuation
Antibiotic Prophylaxis YES ❑ NO ❑ (please tick box)
D.V.T. Prophylaxis YES ❑ NO ❑ (please tick box)
Signature | Bleep No.
Designation
Routine post op care (tick box opposite)
Special written post op instructions

Prepared by: Lloyd Mayers + Fiona Blain (pharmacy) 10 Jan 2011 and updated 16 Feb 2011
Authorised by: NBT Thrombosis Committee 12 Jan 2011
Review date: Jan 2013

(continued)

Appendix 10 *(Continued)*

North Bristol NHS
NHS Trust

Revised VTE Risk Assessment Audit Guide

	Risk assessment	Thrombosis Indicated	Pharmacological			Mechanical		
			Ind	Rx		Ind	Rx	
Audit ..../..../....	Proforma	☐ None	☐	☐	Yes - ??	☐	☐	Yes - ??
Admission ..../..../....	☐ Present	☐ Pharmacological	☐	☐	Enoxaparin	☐	☐	GECS
Planned ☐	☐ Complete	☐ Mechanical	☐	☐	Dabigatran	☐	☐	Pneu
Emerg ☐	☐ O/A	☐ Both	☐	☐	Rivaroxaban			Comp
Ward ______	Thrombosis	☐ Contraindicated	☐	☐	UFH			
Cons ______	☐ Risk ✓	☐ Caution present	☐	☐	Treatment			
Pt ID:	☐ Risk ×		☐	☐	Extended			
	Bleeding	______	☐	☐	Other			
Pt DoB: ..../..../....	☐ Risk ✓	☐ Not recorded	VTE Info: Yes ☐ / No ☐ / Unknown ☐					
Dr grade	☐ Risk ×		Post Op assessment Yes ☐ / No ☐ / N/A ☐					
Audit ..../..../....	Proforma	☐ None	☐	☐	Yes - ??	☐	☐	Yes - ??
Admission ..../..../....	☐ Present	☐ Pharmacological	☐	☐	Enoxaparin	☐	☐	GECS
Planned ☐	☐ Complete	☐ Mechanical	☐	☐	Dabigatran	☐	☐	Pneu
Emerg ☐	☐ O/A	☐ Both	☐	☐	Rivaroxaban			Comp
Ward ______	Thrombosis	☐ Contraindicated	☐	☐	UFH			
Cons ______	☐ Risk ✓	☐ Caution present	☐	☐	Treatment			
Pt ID:	☐ Risk ×		☐	☐	Extended			
	Bleeding	______	☐	☐	Other			
Pt DoB: ..../..../....	☐ Risk ✓	☐ Not recorded	VTE Info: Yes ☐ / No ☐ / Unknown ☐					
Dr grade	☐ Risk ×		Post Op assessment Yes ☐ / No ☐ / N/A ☐					
Audit ..../..../....	Proforma	☐ None	☐	☐	Yes - ??	☐	☐	Yes - ??
Admission ..../..../....	☐ Present	☐ Pharmacological	☐	☐	Enoxaparin	☐	☐	GECS
Planned ☐	☐ Complete	☐ Mechanical	☐	☐	Dabigatran	☐	☐	Pneu
Emerg ☐	☐ O/A	☐ Both	☐	☐	Rivaroxaban			Comp
Ward ______	Thrombosis	☐ Contraindicated	☐	☐	UFH			
Cons ______	☐ Risk ✓	☐ Caution present	☐	☐	Treatment			
Pt ID:	☐ Risk ×		☐	☐	Extended			
	Bleeding	______	☐	☐	Other			
Pt DoB: ..../..../....	☐ Risk ✓	☐ Not recorded	VTE Info: Yes ☐ / No ☐ / Unknown ☐					
Dr grade	☐ Risk ×		Post Op assessment Yes ☐ / No ☐ / N/A ☐					
Audit ..../..../....	Proforma	☐ None	☐	☐	Yes - ??	☐	☐	Yes - ??
Admission ..../..../....	☐ Present	☐ Pharmacological	☐	☐	Enoxaparin	☐	☐	GECS
Planned ☐	☐ Complete	☐ Mechanical	☐	☐	Dabigatran	☐	☐	Pneu
Emerg ☐	☐ O/A	☐ Both	☐	☐	Rivaroxaban			Comp
Ward ______	Thrombosis	☐ Contraindicated	☐	☐	UFH			
Cons ______	☐ Risk ✓	☐ Caution present	☐	☐	Treatment			
Pt ID:	☐ Risk ×		☐	☐	Extended			
	Bleeding	______	☐	☐	Other			
Pt DoB: ..../..../....	☐ Risk ✓	☐ Not recorded	VTE Info: Yes ☐ / No ☐ / Unknown ☐					
Dr grade	☐ Risk ×		Post Op assessment Yes ☐ / No ☐ / N/A ☐					
Audit ..../..../....	Proforma	☐ None	☐	☐	Yes - ??	☐	☐	Yes - ??
Admission ..../..../....	☐ Present	☐ Pharmacological	☐	☐	Enoxaparin	☐	☐	GECS
Planned ☐	☐ Complete	☐ Mechanical	☐	☐	Dabigatran	☐	☐	Pneu
Emerg ☐	☐ O/A	☐ Both	☐	☐	Rivaroxaban			Comp
Ward ______	Thrombosis	☐ Contraindicated	☐	☐	UFH			
Cons ______	☐ Risk ✓	☐ Caution present	☐	☐	Treatment			
Pt ID:	☐ Risk ×		☐	☐	Extended			
	Bleeding	______	☐	☐	Other			
Pt DoB: ..../..../....	☐ Risk ✓	☐ Not recorded	VTE Info: Yes ☐ / No ☐ / Unknown ☐					
Dr grade	☐ Risk ×		Post Op assessment Yes ☐ / No ☐ / N/A ☐					

Prepared by: Lloyd Mayers + Fiona Blain (pharmacy) 10 Jan 2011 and updated 16 Feb 2011
Authorised by: NBT Thrombosis Committee 12 Jan 2011
Review date: Jan 2013

Source: North Bristol NHS Trust and University Hospitals Bristol NHS Foundation Trust. Reproduced with permission.

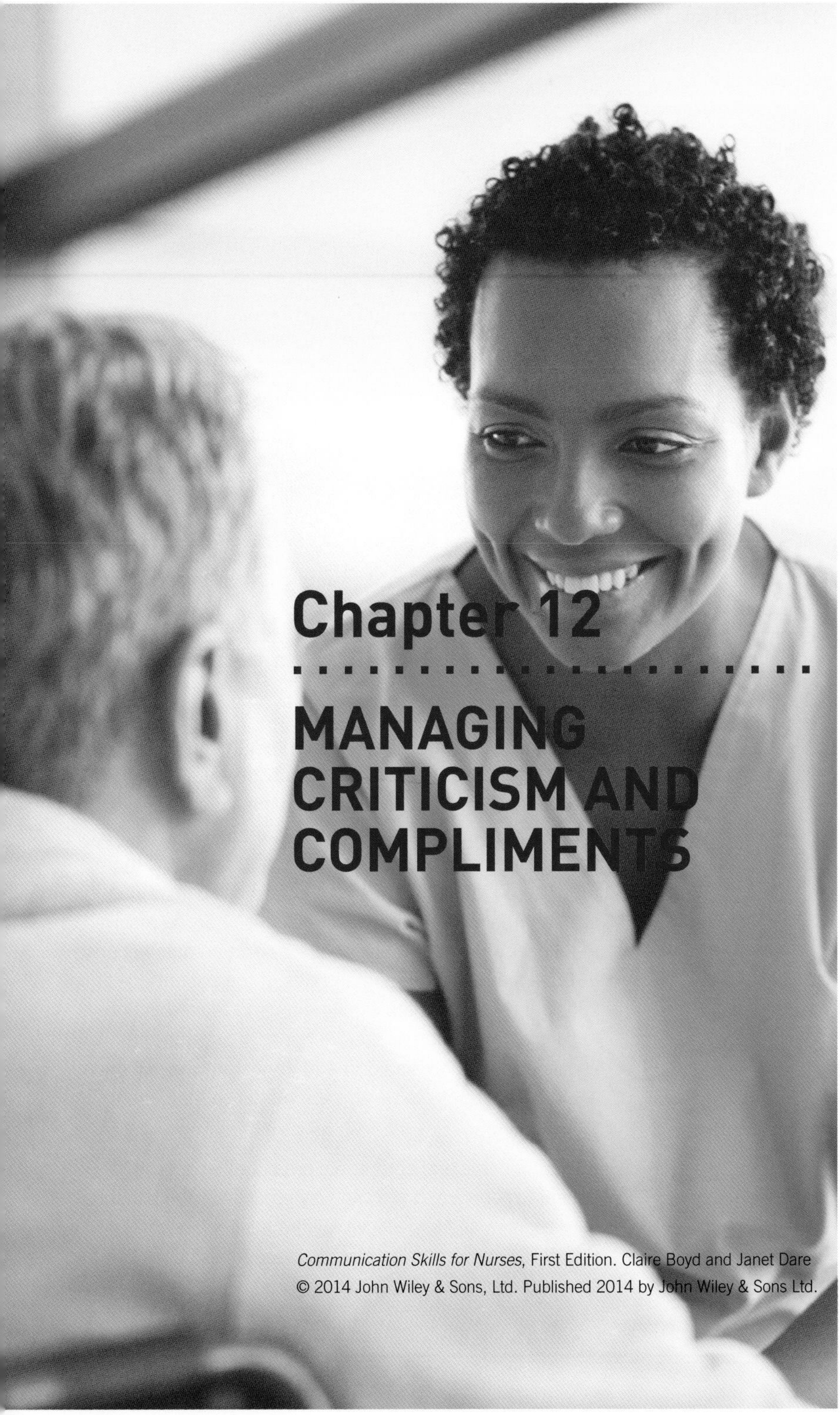

Chapter 12

MANAGING CRITICISM AND COMPLIMENTS

Communication Skills for Nurses, First Edition. Claire Boyd and Janet Dare
© 2014 John Wiley & Sons, Ltd. Published 2014 by John Wiley & Sons Ltd.

LEARNING OUTCOMES

By the end of this chapter you will have an understanding of the complaints procedure and processes in the healthcare environment and what to do when you receive compliments.

CONCERNS AND COMPLAINTS

The NHS Constitution states:

> The NHS commits when mistakes happen, to acknowledge them, apologise, explain what when wrong and put things right quickly and effectively.
>
> Department of Health (2013)

The delivery of exceptional patient health care is at the heart of any NHS trust and care provider. However, sometimes things do go wrong. Having a complaint made against you personally is not a pleasant feeling, but if a patient or service user has a matter that concerns them, they should make their feelings known as soon as possible to a member of staff so that the situation can be resolved in a speedy manner. Many concerns and complaints arise through simple misunderstandings. If the patient does not consider the immediate explanation and related action to satisfactorily address their concern, it will then be escalated to a more senior member of staff who will once again try informally to resolve the matter to the patient's satisfaction.

NOTE: concerns and complaints are not all about the patient experience. It is a two-way process as the patient may become aggressive towards the healthcare worker. Processes and procedures are in place to also deal with this side of things (see later in this chapter).

WHO CAN RAISE A CONCERN/ COMPLAINT?

Anyone who has received treatment from an NHS trust can raise a concern/complaint with that trust. If the person is unable to do so by themselves, a carer, relative or friend can act on their behalf, after obtaining their permission to do so.

ACTIVITY

Activity 12.1

What is the difference between a concern and a complaint?

GLOSSARY

ACT

Advice and Complaints Team.

A patient can raise a concern or complaint about any treatment or service provided by an NHS trust that they (or their friend/relative or carer) have received or are receiving. This does not include dealing with concerns or complaints about other services such as private health care. The number of complaints against doctors in the UK has doubled in the past 5 years, with 8100 complaints in 2012 compared to just under 4000 in 2007 (Triggle 2013).

The NHS monitors all concerns and complaints so that improvements can be made and issues addressed. Concerns/complaints raised with the Advice and Complaints Team (ACT) are added to secure databases to allow trends to be analysed, improvements to be made and subsequent audits to be undertaken. As part of the process the ACT will collect information on whether complainants have a disability, and also their ethnicity and sexual orientation, to ensure that no groups are discriminated against.

CONFIDENTIALITY

All concerns/complaints are treated as strictly confidential. The complainant's health records may be seen by a number of staff while dealing with the concern/complaint, but only on a 'need-to-know' basis. All correspondence about the concern/complaint will be kept separate from a person's health records and will not affect their care or treatment.

THE COMPLAINTS PROCEDURE

The complainant first talks to a staff member who will try to find out what has happened and take any action necessary. This staff member may need to talk to other staff while investigating the concern/complaint.

If the complainant feels that the process and any subsequent escalation to a more senior member of staff has not resolved their concern/complaint, then it will then be communicated to the ACT.

The Advice and Complaints Team will acknowledge receipt and may contact the complainant for any additional information and to agree;

- the complainant's issues,
- any desired outcomes,
- how they want the issue dealt with,
- what action will be taken,
- complexity,
- provisional timescales for resolution.

The ACT will also seek to agree a reasonable response date with the complainant if it is clear from the outset that the team's aim of 25 working days is unlikely to be achieved. This can happen if the concern/complaint involves multiple services and is of a particularly complex nature. If for reasons of complexity or staff availability the resolution takes longer than originally agreed, the ACT will write to the complainant to advise them of this and where possible indicate the new expected response date.

All formal complaints will receive a full explanation in writing from the hospital's Chief Executive. All written complaints must be acknowledged within 3 working days of receipt. Where complaints are addressed to the Chief Executive's Office they will be forwarded to the ACT for acknowledgement.

If the complainant remains dissatisfied with the response to their concern/complaint they have the right to ask the Parliamentary and Health Service Ombudsman to review their case. The Ombudsman is an independent body established to promote improvements in health care by assessing the performance of those who provide services.

BEING OPEN WHEN THINGS GO WRONG

In November 2009 the National Patient Safety Agency (NPSA) published guidelines for NHS organisations that consisted of a set of clear principles describing how NHS staff need to communicate with patients, their families and carers when something goes wrong. This is known as Being Open (www.nrls.nhs.uk/beingopen; see also National Patient Safety Agency 2009).

The Being Open framework maintains that discussing patient safety incidents promptly, fully and compassionately is the best way to support patients and staff when things go wrong. Following the principles of Being Open, evidence from other countries has shown that formal complaints and litigation claims can be reduced.

The framework also describes how boards of NHS organisations need to embed the principles of Being Open to ensure a culture of openness, honesty and transparency is created across the NHS.

One of the requirements of the Being Open Patient Safety Alert (see National Patient Safety Agency 2009) is the need for NHS organisations to introduce senior clinical counsellors, whose role will be to provide specialist advice and support to staff involved in safety incidents.

The Patient Safety Alert detailed key requirements that NHS organisations should follow. They should:

- effectively communicate with patients, their families and carers;
- review and strengthen local policies to ensure they are aligned to the Being Open framework;
- make a board-level public commitment to implement the principles of being Open;
- nominate lead individuals to take responsibility for implementing the local policy within the organisation;
- identify senior clinical counsellors who will monitor and support fellow clinicians;
- raise awareness and understanding of Being Open among staff, patients and the public;
- ensure patient advice services have the information, skills and processes in place to effectively implement Being Open.

Source: National Patient Safety Agency (2009).

THE OMBUDSMAN

Patients have the right to bring their complaint to the Parliamentary and Health Service Ombudsman if they are dissatisfied with the way their complaint was handled at a local level, as stated in the NHS Constitution. Health complaints cover a whole host of issues, such as clinical care treatment, funding and medication.

Figure 12.1 shows subject keywords assigned to health complaints from the period of 2009–2010 by the NHS in England. It can be seen that the largest number of complaints revolved around clinical care and treatment. Figure 12.2 shows complaint handling subject keywords assigned to health complaints whereby 'poor explanation' made up the second largest group of complaints (after 'other' non-specific complaints) received in the Ombudsman's office by the NHS in England 2009–2010 (House of Commons 2010).

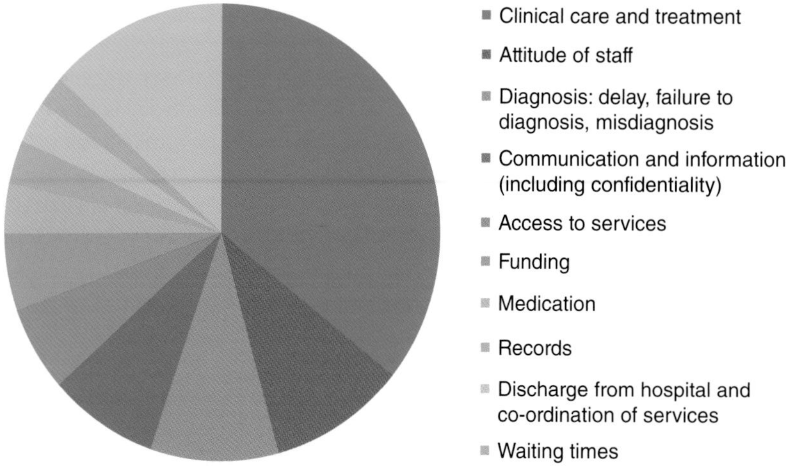

Figure 12.1 Subject keywords assigned to health complaints. The size of each pie slice represents the number of complaints.

Source: House of Commons (2010).

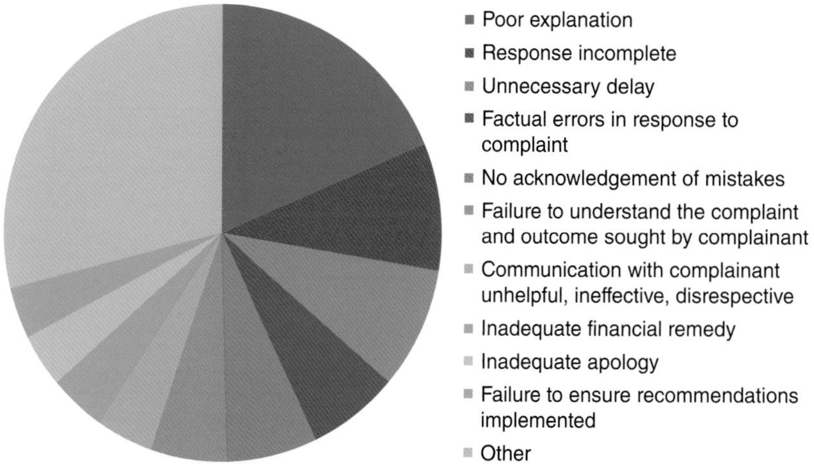

Figure 12.2 Complaint handling subject keywords assigned to health complaints. The size of each pie slice represents the number of complaints.

Source: House of Commons (2010). Reproduced with permission of Parliamentary and Health Service Ombudsman.

The Ombudsman's department receives many thousands of enquiries about the NHS every year. Each one is assessed to find a way of resolving the issues. If local resolution has been completed, this assessment involves checking the quality of the NHS response to the complaint, testing the evidence supporting the response and comparing any clinical issues against relevant accepted good practice using the Ombudsman's team of independent clinical advisors.

The Ombudsman's complaint-handling process can be seen in Figure 12.3. It should be noted that at any stage

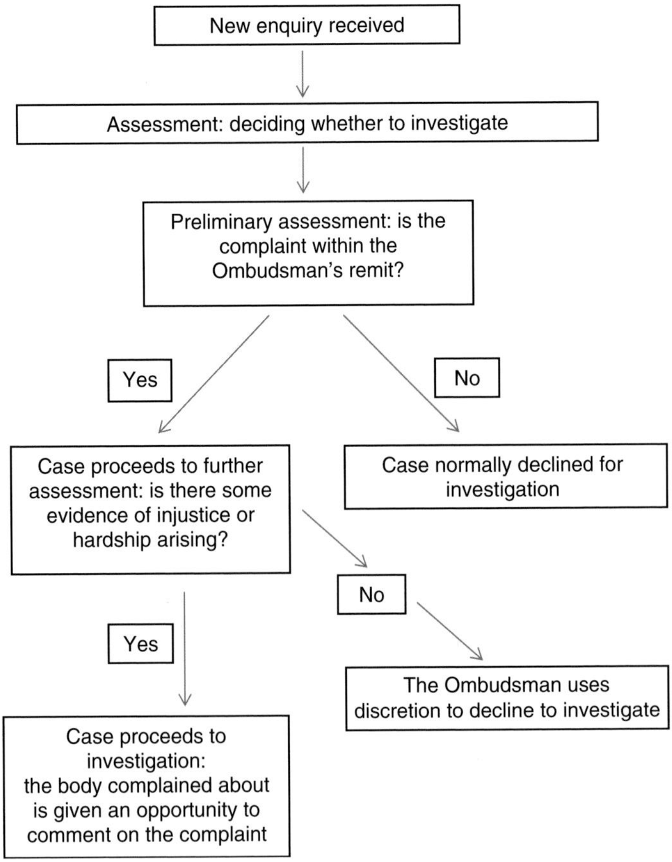

Figure 12.3 The Ombudsman's complaint-handling process.

Source: adapted from House of Commons (2010).

of the assessment process the Ombudsman's office may attempt resolution through intervention.

OMBUDSMAN COMPLAINT, REVIEW AND OUTCOME

Below is an example of the type of complaint investigated by the Ombudsman and the outcome, taken from *Listening and Learning: the Ombudsman's Review of Complaint Handling by the NHS in England 2009–10* (House of Commons 2010).

Mr C and his Son J's Story

J, aged 7, has cerebral palsy and requires the constant use of a wheelchair. He is a growing child, and regularly outgrows his wheelchairs, which are provided by Plymouth Teaching Primary Care Trust (PCT) Wheelchair Services.

J and his parents experienced substantial delays, having to wait several months before the PCT acted on requests at first for an initial wheelchair assessment and later for adjustments to the chair or replacements. Between March 2005, when J was first referred for a wheelchair, and January 2009 he had to wait around 8 months on three separate occasions for an appropriate wheelchair or for adjustments to be made so that his wheelchair was suitable for him to use. These delays meant that J was forced to use a wheelchair that was too small for him, or that his family had to carry him or push him in a pushchair.

Mr C complained about the delays, but, although he received replies from the PCT, the service the family received did not improve. He decided to take the case to the Ombudsman, and an investigation into the situation was launched on his and his son's behalf.

What the Investigation Found

The delays J had experienced were excessive and had caused him and his family significant distress and inconvenience. Having either no wheelchair at all, or using one that was unsuitable, affected J's schooling and he had to cope with further attention being drawn to his disability among his peers.

It was clear that the service the PCT were providing did not address the fact that children using wheelchairs will regularly require assistance to either adjust them, or obtain new ones without delay. In total, J had spent more than two of his 7 years waiting for wheelchairs, or for adjustments to his wheelchairs. The Ombudsman accepted that the PCT had attempted to improve their service but it was clear that this had not specifically helped J or his family. Instead, the failure to address the issues in Mr C's complaint had compounded their frustration and distress.

What Happened Next

The PCT apologised to Mr and Mrs C for the injustice their family had suffered as a result of both the original delays and the failure to respond appropriately to their complaint. They told the Ombudsman that they had reduced the average waiting times for paediatric wheelchair service users to 8 weeks, and were working to reduce this even further.

The Ombudsman recommended that the PCT make a payment of £5000 in compensation to Mr and Mrs C, which could be used to fund a new wheelchair for their son.

DEALING WITH AGGRESSION IN THE HEALTHCARE ENVIRONMENT

NOTE: as a student nurse, assistant practitioner or health care assistant, you should always refer a complainant to a more senior member of staff. Should a patient become aggressive while relaying their complaint to you in person there are certain strategies that you can use to de-escalate the situation.

ACTIVITY

Activity 12.2

You are a newly qualified nurse assigned to the out-patient clinic. A male patient has been waiting for 40 minutes in a packed waiting room, waiting to be seen, and has complained to you about this. You have apologised for the delay and have offered to find out when he will be seen. However, the patient now becomes aggressive. What strategies do you use to reduce his agression?

Don't forget to ensure that you document any incident of aggression and inform your manager.

DEALING WITH DIFFICULT TELEPHONE CALLS

If you receive a telephone call that develops into abuse and insult from the caller:

- as positively as possible interrupt the conversation firmly;
- advise the caller that you wish to assist them but you will end the call if the caller does not stop using intimidating/threatening/abusive or aggressive language.

If the caller continues to be intimidating:

- politely advise the caller that you are terminating the conversation and place your handset in its cradle;
- inform the nurse in charge, supervisor or manager of the incident.

If the caller phones back:

- remind the caller that you expect them to speak to you courteously and that if this does not happen the call will be terminated;

- try to assist the caller if possible;
- if the abusive behaviour persists, confirm with the caller their telephone number (if you do not have it already).

Complete the necessary documentation, detailing as much as possible about the incident. If you are distressed by the call or have concerns about handling future calls from the same individual, inform your manager, as help will be available.

THE NHS FRIENDS AND FAMILY TEST

The NHS wants to ensure that patients have the best possible experience of care. The **Friends and Family Test** is a way of gathering feedback about this experience and helping to drive improvement in hospital services. When patients receive care as an inpatient or in an emergency department they will be given the opportunity to give you feedback by answering a simple question about their experience. The results provide a way for everyone to easily compare NHS hospitals to know where they themselves and their family members can get the best possible care. The information also gives the NHS invaluable information on what patients think of services, which can be used to help make improvements if required.

In short, the NHS wishes to acquire information of the patient experience regardless of whether the feedback is positive, negative or indifferent. The results are rapidly analysed to see if any action is required, and they are published so that hospitals can be compared with each other. The results are published in hospital annual reports and quality accounts, and can be viewed on the NHS Choices website (www.nhs.uk).

Patients can still pass their compliments or complaints to the hospital in the normal way, so this feedback does not replace the existing compliments or complaints procedure. The Friends and Family Test is in addition to this normal procedure. When they are discharged, or within the 48 hours that follow, patients are asked to answer the following question:

> How likely are you to recommend our ward/ emergency department to friends and family if they needed similar care or treatment?

They will be invited to respond to the question by choosing one of six options, ranging from 'extremely likely' to 'extremely unlikely'. It is very important that the patient then explains why they gave their answer by answering any follow-up questions.

Patients may be asked to answer the question before going home, or invited to do so by returning a postcard, by phone or on the hospital's website. Patient's answers are anonymous, and their details will not be passed on to anyone, so they can say exactly what they thought about their care. A member of the patient's family or a friend is welcome to help the patient complete their answer to the question if they are unable to do so alone. Patients do not have to respond to the question, but if they do the feedback will provide valuable information to the hospital to help ensure that all patients have the best possible experience of care.

COMPLIMENTS

As a nurse or assistant practitioner you are expected to keep a portfolio as evidence of your continuing professional development. This should include sections on reflection in practice and all the study sessions you have attended. You may be asked to bring this with you when attending interviews. It is therefore considered good practice to include in this portfolio evidence of any patients' complaints, and how you dealt with them. Do not forget to include 'thank you' letters and cards from grateful patients who have complimented you on your care. Blow your own trumpet! After all, the patient went out of their way to tell the hospital how good they thought your care skills were.

TEST YOUR KNOWLEDGE

1 What is the difference between a concern and a complaint?
2 What does ACT stand for?
3 What are single most common set of complaint handling subject keywords assigned to health complaints?
4 Who published the Being Open guidelines in November 2009?
5 What is the name of the test used to acquire feedback from patients (or their family) about their care experience?
6 Where should you keep evidence of compliments received from patients?

KEY POINTS

- **Who can raise a concern or complaint**
- **Knowing the difference between a concern and a complaint**
- **The complaints procedure**
- **The importance of Being Open**
- **The Ombudsman's complaint-handling process**
- **Dealing with aggression in the healthcare environment**
- **The NHS Friends and Family Test**
- **What to do with your compliments**

Bibliography

Department of Health (2013) *The Handbook to the NHS Constitution*. Department of Health, London.

House of Commons (2010) *Listening and Learning: the Ombudsman's Review of Complaint Handling by the NHS in England 2009–10*. The Stationery Office, London.

North Bristol NHS Trust (2010) *Concerns, Complaints and Compliments Booklet.* North Bristol NHS Trust, Bristol.

National Patient Safety Agency (2009) *Being Open – Communicating with Patients, Their Families and Carers Following a Patient Safety Incident.* Patient Safety Alert NPSA/2009/PSA003. National Patient Safety Agency, London.

Triggle, N. (2013) Complaints about doctors 'double in 5 years'. BBC News, Health. www.bbc.co.uk/news/health-24534273.

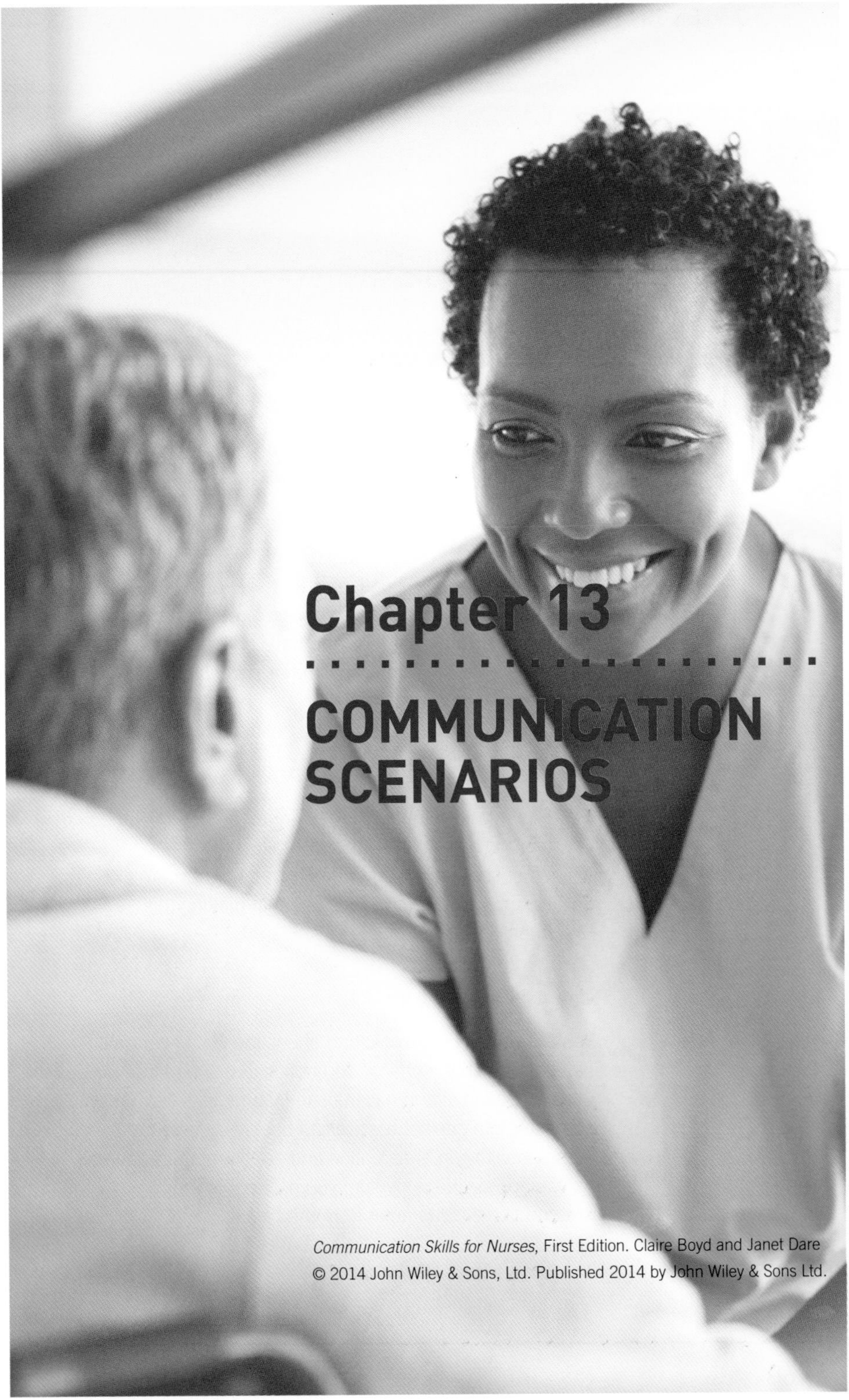

Chapter 13

COMMUNICATION SCENARIOS

Communication Skills for Nurses, First Edition. Claire Boyd and Janet Dare
© 2014 John Wiley & Sons, Ltd. Published 2014 by John Wiley & Sons Ltd.

LEARNING OUTCOMES

By the end of this chapter, having read the communication scenarios, you will be able to feel more confident with your own communication skills in your work area.

Below are example scenarios relating to communication problems which you may encounter in the healthcare setting. Think about how you would manage each of these scenarios. Suggested answers to scenarios 1–8 can be found in the Answer section at the back of the book.

SCENARIO ONE

You are looking after a patient whose speech has been badly affected by a stroke (dysphasia). You have cared for her on several occasions and have built up a good relationship. You are familiar with her speech and can communicate effectively with her. One morning she confides in you that she is getting frustrated with other members of staff.

1. How would you approach the other members of the team to highlight this patient's difficulties?
2. What suggestions for improvement might you make?
3. How can you involve the patient in making this improvement?

SCENARIO TWO

You are working in a clinic and check the list for who will be attending that morning. You notice that one of the patients due to attend has the same name as a well-known character in a current best-selling book. You hear the person booking in at reception and go to introduce yourself. As you approach the person, you notice that they are dressed like the character from the book.

1. What action will you take?

SCENARIO THREE

You are working on a very busy orthopaedic ward when the phone rings. On answering the call you find that the person at the other end of the line does not have English as their first language. You find the person very difficult to understand and do not know what they require.

1 How do you overcome this barrier to effective communication?

SCENARIO FOUR

It is 2.15 on a Friday afternoon. Susan Jones, a medical secretary, is working at her desk when she is approached by Christine Brown, a staff nurse who looks after the surgical clinics in the Out-patients' Department. They have not met before.

Christine asks Susan where Mr Gregory, the consultant surgeon, is. Apparently, he is due to be running an extra waiting list initiative clinic but he hasn't turned up. The clinic was due to begin at 2 p.m. and patients have been arriving since 1.30 p.m. There are 12 patients due at the clinic.

Susan is not Mr Gregory's secretary – she has the day off – but Susan discovers that Mr Gregory is working at another hospital, as he normally does on Friday afternoons. When he is contacted, Mr Gregory says he didn't know that this extra clinic had been arranged. He had agreed to run three extra clinics but didn't know that the dates had been booked. There was nothing in his diary.

Mr Gregory says he will be there as soon as he can but that it probably won't be before 3.30 or 3.45 p.m. It could be later. If patients care to wait, he will see them when he arrives. He is also concerned to discover that the remaining two extra clinics are due to be held on the two following Friday afternoons, and he is already booked up with other patients on both Fridays. Either these patients or the patients at the waiting list initiative clinic will need to have their appointments cancelled.

First look at this situation from the point of view of Christine, the staff nurse, and answer the following questions.

1. Who is your customer?
2. What help did you expect Susan to give you?
3. Once it is known that Mr Gregory cannot be at the clinic until 3.30 p.m. at the earliest, what should the patients be told and what action needs to be taken?
4. Should you keep the patients informed as the afternoon progresses? If so, what information should they be given and how often?

Now look at it from the point of view of a patient and answer the following questions.

1. What was your initial impression of the hospital?
2. Once it is known that Mr Gregory could not be in the clinic until 3.30 p.m. at the earliest, what information should you have been given?
3. Should you have been kept informed as the afternoon progressed? If so, what information would you have wanted and how often?
4. What else would you like to have been done for you?
5. How can this problem be avoided in the future?

SCENARIO FIVE

Mohammed is visiting his wife in hospital following her minor operation. She has dementia and cannot fully understand what is happening to her, which makes both of them feel anxious. He hovers around the nurses' station, hoping to speak to someone about her progress, but they all seem too busy. Eventually a nurse looks up and in a rather dismissive way asks him what he wants. The nurse answers his questions but appears distracted, saying his wife is 'doing as well as one would expect'. He then asks her if she is being given a halal diet and is told, 'I expect so, if that's what she requested'.

1. List different reasons why Mohammed needs to communicate.
2. How could the nurse improve her communication skills?

SCENARIO SIX

As a student nurse you have recently commenced working on a placement looking after older people with dementia. Karen, a healthcare assistant, has worked on the ward for many years and you overhear her speaking to the patients as if they were children and referring to them as 'love' and 'sweetheart'. When you speak to her about this she informs you that they are like children and are always spilling food and being incontinent.

1 What do you think about Karen's communication skills and why?

SCENARIO SEVEN

You see on Facebook that someone you know has written that they have had a really bad day at work because of a certain person, who is actually named.

1 What should you do in this situation?

SCENARIO EIGHT

During a tutorial you are listening to a lecturer but you are finding it very hard to concentrate because the person sitting next to you sending and receiving lots of text messages, and his phone bleeping constantly.

1 What should you do?

You will encounter many situations like those above. As a qualified nurse, you will adhere to the Nursing and Midwifery Council's Code of Conduct (Nursing and Midwifery Council 2008), a set of standards and the foundation of good nursing and midwifery practice.

TEST YOUR KNOWLEDGE

Suggested answers to scenarios 1–8 can be found in the Answer section at the back of the book.

KEY POINT

- **Communication scenarios**

Bibliography

Nursing and Midwifery Council (2008) *The Code: Standards of Conduct, Performance and Ethics for Nurses and Midwives*. NMC, London; www.nmc-uk.org/code.

Royal College of Nursing (2010) *The Principles of Nursing Practice: Principles and Measures Consultation*. Royal College of Nursing, London; www.rcn.org.uk/__data/assets/pdf_file/0007/349549/003875.pdf.

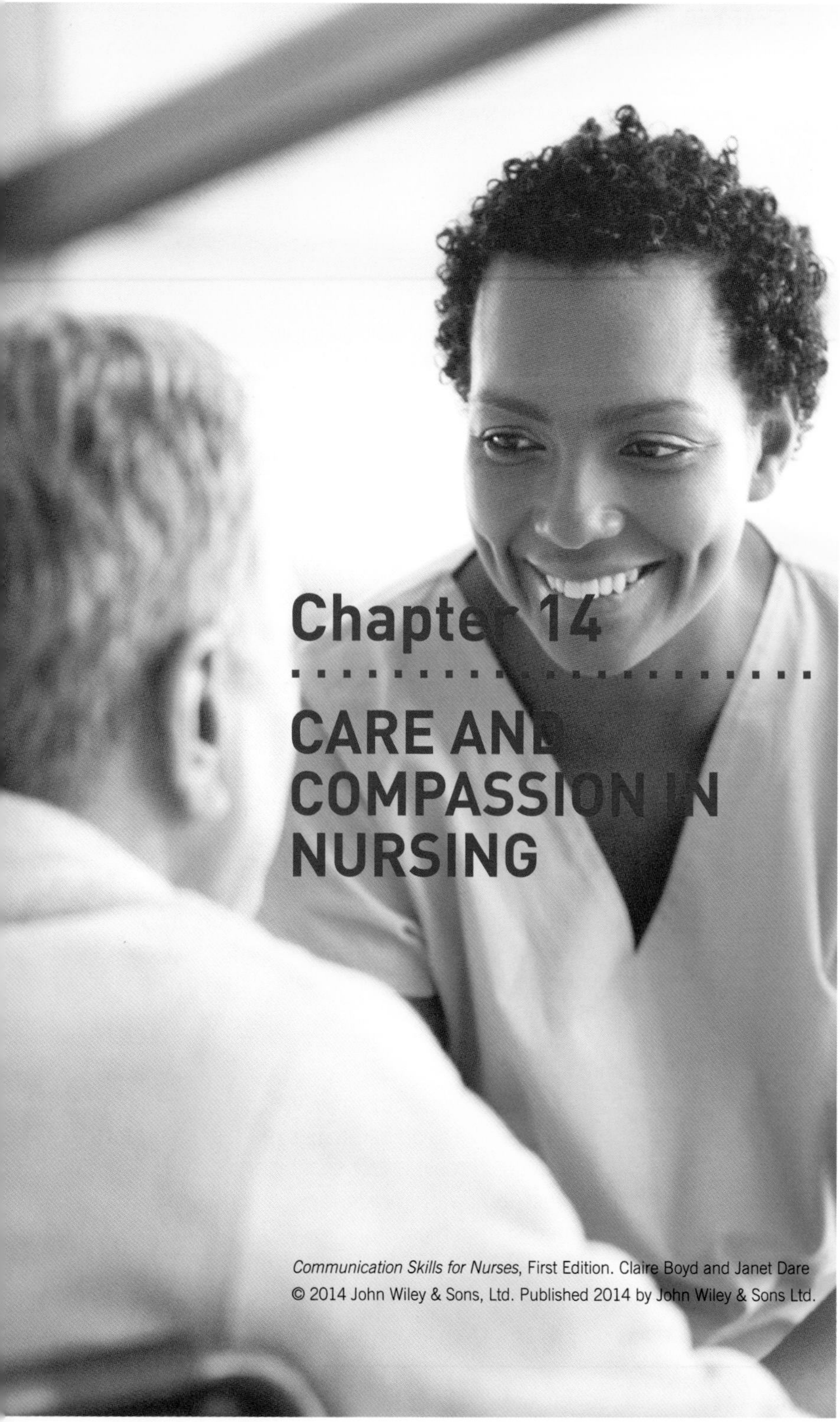

Chapter 14

CARE AND COMPASSION IN NURSING

Communication Skills for Nurses, First Edition. Claire Boyd and Janet Dare
© 2014 John Wiley & Sons, Ltd. Published 2014 by John Wiley & Sons Ltd.

LEARNING OUTCOMES

By the end of this chapter you will have an understanding of the meaning of care and compassion in nursing.

One of the most important reports in the history of the NHS is what has become known as the Francis Report (Mid Staffordshire NHS Foundation Trust Public Inquiry 2013). This report investigated events at Mid Staffordshire NHS Foundation Trust. It is littered with accounts of bad nursing practice, such as:

- staff being rude to patients and visitors,
- meals being placed out of sick patients' reach,
- staff being too busy to toilet patients,
- staff being too busy to change soiled bed sheets,
- patients not being given their prescribed medication,
- patients becoming extremely dehydrated due to not being given water to drink,
- the list goes on.

Unfortunately, examples of poor nursing practice can be observed across all care settings, and not just in hospitals. The Royal College of Nursing (RCN), in its response to the Francis Report (Royal College of Nursing 2013), tells us that poor practice is not just about delivering poor care to patients. It is also about not doing enough to prevent poor care in the first place. The response also states:

> The RCN believes that the NHS often sets up good people to do bad things; through constant change, chronic under-staffing and unrelenting pressure, staff have kindness and compassion eroded from them.
>
> Royal College of Nursing (2013).

CARE AND COMPASSION

Addressing the care and compassion issue in health care has instigated the RCN to launch a campaign to show the 'skill and compassion' of today's nurses, as well as exploring the reasons behind failures in care (see the This is Nursing website; Royal College of Nursing 2012).

This campaign, developed jointly with the Royal College of Nursing, The Nursing and Midwifery Council and the Department of Health, has produced the Principles of Nursing Practice, which tell us what patients, colleagues, families and carers can expect from nursing. These principles are reproduced in Table 14.1.

Table 14.1 The principles of nursing practice

A	**Nurses and nursing staff treat everyone in their care with dignity and humanity – they understand their individual needs, show compassion and sensitivity, and provide care in a way that respects all people equally.**
B	**Nurses and nursing staff take responsibility for the care they provide and answer for their own judgements and actions – they carry out these actions in a way that is agreed with their patients, and their families and carers of their patients, and in a way that meets the requirements of their professional bodies and the law.**
C	**Nurses and nursing staff manage risk, are vigilant about risk, and help to keep everyone safe in the places they receive health care.**
D	**Nurses and nursing staff provide and promote care that puts people at the centre, involves patients, service users, their families and their carers in decisions and helps them make informed choices about their treatment and care.**
E	**Nurses and nursing staff are at the heart of the communication process: they assess, record and report on treatment and care, handle information sensitively and confidentially, deal with complaints effectively, and are conscientious in reporting the things they are concerned about.**
F	**Nurses and nursing staff have an up-to-date knowledge and skills, and use these with intelligence, insight and understanding in line with the needs of each individual in their care.**

(continued)

Table 14.1 *(Continued)*

G	**Nurses and nursing staff work closely with their own team and with other professionals, making sure patients' care and treatment is co-ordinated, is of a high standard and has the best possible outcome.**
H	**Nurses and nursing staff lead by example, develop themselves and other staff, and influence the way care is given in a manner that is open and responds to individual needs.**

From Royal College of Nursing (2010). Reproduced with permission of Royal College of Nursing.

GLOSSARY

Compassion

A feeling of distress and pity for the suffering or misfortune of others. This often includes the desire to alleviate it.

The Department of Health and the NHS Commissioning Board have developed a consultation/discussion paper (see Department of Health and NHS Commissioning Board 2012) to emphasise values and behaviours in the NHS, public health and in social care. These values are known as the six Cs (Box 14.1).

Box 14.1

The culture of compassionate care: the six Cs

Care
Compassion
Competence
Communication
Courage
Commitment

From Department of Health and NHS Commissioning Board (2012).

If you go to any care setting in the NHS – into care homes, healthcare clinics and individual's own homes – you will see abundant examples of excellent care and compassion given to those in need. Unfortunately it is the relatively few cases, often shocking in their brutality, that are publicised in the media.

PATIENTS' COMPLAINTS

Chapter 12 looked at the complaints procedure and examples investigated by the Parliamentary and Health Service Ombudsman.

The Patients Association, a charitable organisation that aims to tackle poor care and the causes of poor care, published their report entitled *We've Been Listening, Have You Been Learning?* in 2011, and gave the four most frequent complaints received by The Patients Association, from patients. What do you think they were?

ACTIVITY

Activity 14.1

Name the four most frequent complaints received by The Patients Association from patients.

How many of you have groaned when you have looked at your weekly timetable to see that you have yet another communications lecture or seminar! But as the number one complaint from patients is concerned with communications, it is quite obvious we are not getting this aspect right!

THE FRANCIS REPORT

The Francis Report looked at the 'appalling care' received by the people of Stafford during the period 2005–2008 by the Mid Staffordshire NHS Foundation Trust. Robert Francis QC and his team collected over 1 million pages of documentary material, gathered information from 250 witnesses and undertook 139 days of oral hearings. From this 290 recommendations were produced. We will now look at a very small part of the Francis Report; those aspects relationing to communication (see Mid Staffordshire NHS Foundation Trust Public Inquiry 2013).

Recommendation 271 Communication with patients and those closest to them requires staff to have ready access to the relevant information, and the time to impart it. This requires good record-keeping, proper handovers and a caring attitude, promoting the easy recall of particular patients and their problems. Provision of information should not be treated as a nuisance to be fitted in when convenient to staff. It is an intrinsic and vital part of the process of treatment. Patients are entitled to information enabling them to judge the progress of their treatment and to make relevant decisions about it. Those closest to them may be able to assist in the assessment of the best interests of those who cannot make decisions for themselves. Treatment and care are matters in which the patient should be involved in partnership, along with those that he or she aggress to be involved.

Recommendation 274 Being in hospital can be a lonely experience. The simple reassurance that some other human being cares about the patient, and identifies with what he or she is going through, is tremendously important. The relative of one patient remarked:

> It was lack of anything; compassion; nobody ever came in to see Mum and just say: how are you [name]? Which my Mum used to love. That was the whole thing about the home, they would call her by name. She loved it. She liked a bit of fuss actually, if I am honest. But no, no compassion whatsoever.

Recommendation 275 Such compassion can be shown by any member of staff: it merely requires thoughtfulness and recognition of the human needs of others, qualities which surely every member of a hospital's staff should share.

Recommendation 276 One elderly but very lively patient who was a retired nurse herself told me:

> [A member of the nursing staff] who was in training doing the university course, I think, and she was doing a little spell on the ward, and on my first day she came and sat and chatted with me and talked about my experiences and my problem, and I enjoyed that, but that was the only time while I was in there that anybody came and talked to me.

Recommendation 293 The manner in which staff communicated information could also pay insufficient regard to the patient's condition. I heard from the daughter of a patient who was partially deaf. She recalls that staff took the patient's failure to respond as indication of her dementia as opposed to a hearing problem. Another family told me about the language used to communicate with their mother and that the nurse was patronising, referring to her mother as having been 'naughty', affording her little dignity and respect.

Recommendation 294 Casual remarks can often cause distress. One patient's daughter told me:

> We didn't see anyone treated as an individual. We were a commodity to be shifted through the system as quickly as possible. That is the feeling you got, observing 24/7. There is an example of that – a throw-away comment by the doctor to us: 'it is amazing, they normally fade away'.

Recommendation 300 It is an essential part of the care of any patient that adequate information is handed over from shift to shift and between different clinical teams and departments. I heard of occasions when relatives were told that a patient had been discharged when he or she was still being treated as an inpatient. In others, the hospital social services department had not been made aware that a patient required an assessment, and a patient assessed as being at high risk of falls on one ward was transferred to another ward without the information being passed on. A considerable number of families told me that there was a lack of communication across the hospital and there was a failure to take a 'joined-up' approach to patient's care. Families also told me that they do not believe that nursing staff are undertaking a sufficient handover between shifts, as staff coming onto a shift appeared to have little knowledge of their relative or the significant events of the day.

Recommendation 332 The daughter of another patient has not got over the fact that she unwittingly spent the morning on which her father died preparing for his return home when his discharge was cancelled without her being informed because he had contracted *C. difficile*.

> Well, nobody told me that, otherwise I would not have wasted my time on the following morning, the day that my father passed away, re-organising his bedroom at home. I could have been with him. That is terrible.

TEST YOUR KNOWLEDGE

1. Name the six components of the culture of compassionate care.
2. Go and ***be*** the nurse in number 276 of the Francis report.

KEY POINTS

- Care and compassion in nursing
- The culture of compassionate care
- The Principles of Nursing Practice
- Patient complaints
- The Francis Report

Bibliography

Department of Health (2013a) *Caldicott Review: Information Governance in the Health and Care System*. Department of Health, London.

Department of Health (2013b) *Delivering High Quality, Effective, Compassionate Care: Developing the Right People with the Right Skills and the Right Values – a Mandate from the Government to Health Education England: April 2013 to March 2015*. Department of Health, London.

Department of Health and NHS Commissioning Board (2012) *Developing the Culture of Compassionate Care: Creating a New Vision for Nurses, Midwives and Care-givers*. Consultation/discussion paper. Department of Health, London.

Dreaper, J. (2012) Campaign to show 'skill and compassion' of nurses. BBC News, Health, 17 September.

Mid Staffordshire NHS Foundation Trust Public Inquiry (2013) *Report of the Mid Staffordshire NHS Foundation Trust Public Inquiry; Executive Summary* (Chair: R. Francis). Stationery Office, London.

Royal College of Nursing (2010) *The Principles of Nursing Practice: Principles and Measures Consultation*. Royal College of Nursing, London; www.rcn.org.uk/__data/assets/pdf_file/0007/349549/003875.pdf.

Royal College of Nursing (2012) This is nursing. http://thisisnursing.rcn.org.uk/.

Royal College of Nursing (2013) *Mid Staffordshire NHS Foundation Trust Public Inquiry Report – Response of the Royal College of Nursing*. Royal College of Nursing, London.

The Patients Association (2011) *We've Been Listening, Have You Been Learning?* www.patients-association.com.

Willis Commission (2012) *Quality with Compassion; the Future of Nursing Education*. Report of the Willis Commission on Nursing Education. RCN on behalf of the independent Willis Commission on Nursing Education, London.

Answers to Activities and Test Your Knowledge

CHAPTER 1

Chapter 1 Test Your Knowledge

1. A communication model is a process in which information is channelled then imparted by a sender to a receiver through a medium. When the receiver gets the information they decode the message and may give the sender feedback.
2. The linear model, originally known as 'a mathematical model of communication'.
3. Non-verbal communication methods such as gestures, eye contact, use of silence, positioning, facial expression and body language.

CHAPTER 2

Activity 2.1

The doctor has assumed an adult state to tell the patient about the health risks of smoking. In response, the patient was probably in a rebellious child state and was trying to control the situation. The doctor would have responded in an adult state and did not give the reassurance needed by the patient. A nurturing parent ego would have been more appropriate for the doctor to use in this situation.

Chapter 2 Test Your Knowledge

1. The aim of transactional analysis is to find out what state of mind or 'ego' state started the communication process, which one responded and how this affects the relationship of the two people involved.
2. Parent, adult and child
3. This is any transaction where the person being spoken to refuses the ego state that they are assigned by the first speaker.

CHAPTER 3

Activity 3.1

1. Explaining diagnosis, investigations and treatment to the patient
2. Communicating with relatives

Communication Skills for Nurses, First Edition. Claire Boyd and Janet Dare
© 2014 John Wiley & Sons, Ltd. Published 2014 by John Wiley & Sons Ltd.

3 Communicating effectively with health-care and other professionals
4 Involving a patient in decision-making
5 Helping with 'breaking bad news'
6 Dealing with anxious patients/relatives
7 Giving information and instructions on discharge
8 Seeking informed consent
9 Giving health-promotion information or outlining risk factors
10 Introducing yourself/your role to the patient, service user, etc.

Activity 3.2

Jargon, terminology or abbreviation	Meaning
proof of concept	pilot study
efficiency savings and disinvestment	cuts
let's take this discussion off-line	let's talk about this later
STAT	immediately
C-section	Caesarean section
CAT/CT scan	computerised axial tomography scan
BP	blood pressure
FX	bone fracture
ABG	arterial blood gas
vitals	vital signs
MRI	magnetic resonance imaging
claudication	limping caused by a reduction in blood supply to leg
AF	atrial fibrillation
WN	well nourished
TPR	temperature, pulse and respirations
W/C	wheelchair
O2	oxygen
PCA	patient-controlled analgesia
PC	after meals
SB	spina bifida
NIDDM	non-insulin-dependent diabetes mellitus
SS	social services
NG	naso-gastric
GB	gallbladder
Na	sodium
PCN	penicillin
MS	multiple sclerosis
PE	pulmonary embolism
PO	by mouth
SZ	seizure
PRN	*pro re nata*, as required
HX	history
NKA	no known abnormalities
ICP	intracranial pressure
IHD	ischaemic heart disease

BSA	body surface area
SOB	short of breath
C/O	complains of
BI	brain injury
Ca	calcium
CL	cleft lip
BE	barium enema
BG	blood glucose
DOA	dead on arrival or date of admission
COAD	chronic obstructive airways disease
CSF	cerebrospinal fluid
BO	bowels opened
DVT	deep-vein thrombosis
CP	chest pain
MAOIs	monoamine oxidase inhibitors (a category of antidepressant drugs)

Activity 3.3

1 Information missed, patients missed out, poor nurse communication and handover not received from the named nurse
2 Distractions, including noise, interruptions and inattention of staff
3 Lack of confidentiality including no privacy at the nurses' station; relatives in close proximity
4 No handover at the start of the shift, and not receiving any handover at all

Chapter 3 Test Your Knowledge

1 …good-quality health care.
2 verbal, non-verbal, written, visual
3 The vague patient, the scared patient, the guarded paranoid patient, the talkative patient, the manic patient, the angry patient, the demanding patient, the dying patient, the sad patient, the dramatic patient, the anxious patient, the restless patient, the rambling patient, the depressed patient, the patient in pain
4 confidential, uninterrupted, brief, accurate, named nurse
5 SBAR is a communication tool used to impart information in a précised and focused manner; the acronym stands for Situation, Background, Assessment and Recommendations.
6 Abbreviations may be misunderstood by professionals, carers and patients.

CHAPTER 4

Activity 4.1

A customer is an individual at the receiving end of a service. This could be a positive or negative experience.

Activity 4.2

1 Referring to patients as customers suggests a more business-like, impersonal relationship. Serving

customers means meeting the needs and desires of the individual. This could include allowing a patient to smoke a cigarette, but is this in their best interests? This would be poor patient care.

2 Serving customers implies more of a monetary goal than a caring one.

3 In a hospital that is run as a business the driving force behind decision making may not be what is best for the patient.

Chapter 4 Test Your Knowledge

1 The difference between a customer and a patient is that a customer expects good service and is in a position to demand it. Hospital 'customers' are very different for one important reason: they don't want to be there.

2 The way you present yourself, how you look and how you act is important in establishing individual's trust in you.

3 Visual: think about your body language and facial expressions.
Appearance: uniform, tidy hair, clean short nails, no nail polish.
Verbal communication: do not use jargon or abbreviations; think about the tone of your voice and how you address your customer; be polite, smile.
Environment: clean, tidy, not cluttered, think about health and safety aspects, such as spillages on floor, wires, fire exits.

CHAPTER 5

Chapter 5 Test Your Knowledge

1 Interpersonal skills are skills that are exhibited when nurses demonstrate their abilities to use evidence-based and theory-based styles of communication with their patients and colleagues.

2 Effective communication, anger management, conflict resolution, assertiveness, teamwork

CHAPTER 6

Activity 6.1

Examples include having clear team objectives, good communication skills, regular and effective team meetings, role clarity, shared team commitment and integration between team members.

Chapter 6 Test Your Knowledge

1 A team is defined as a small number of people with complementary skills who are committed to a common purpose, performance goals and approach for which they are mutually accountable.

2 Efficient means productive working with minimum wasted effort; "doing things right". Effective means producing the desired result; "doing the right thing".

3 The lack of shared learning between health-care professionals; i.e. they are all educated independently.
4 Can depend on where the student works: physiotherapist, occupational therapist, doctor/GP, nurse/district nurse, speech and language therapist, social worker, chiropodist, dietician.

CHAPTER 7

Activity 7.2

The individual will certainly feel anxious about not being able to communicate their feelings, and this might lead to a sense of loss of control, and frustration. They might not be able to warn the nurse when or where they have pain during the dressing change. They may feel isolated from other patients and staff, and find it difficult to attract attention when they need to communicate.

Chapter 7 Test Your Knowledge

Potential barriers: the environment; physical distractions, e.g. noise; not speaking the same language; accents; jargon; stereotyping or making assumptions; emotion/feelings; pain; muddled messages, whether verbal or written; not listening; different culture; people with disabilities (deafness, blindness, or mental or physical disabilities).

CHAPTER 8

Chapter 8 Test Your Knowledge

1 Active listening is a structured form of listening and responding that focuses the attention on the speaker.
2 Forces people to listen attentively to others; avoids misunderstandings as individuals have to confirm that they have understood what has been saidl helps during conflicts as solutions may be more likely to be found if both parties are actively listening.
3 Face the speaker. Maintain eye contact. Respond appropriately to show your understanding, validating statements and making statements of support. Try to minimise external distractions: give the speaker your full attention. Try to minimise internal distractions: listen to what is being said and stay focused. Focus solely on the person speaking to you and what they are saying. Avoid letting the speaker know how you handled a similar situation. Show good manners: even if the speaker is making a complaint about you, allow them to finish before defending yourself. Engage yourself: ask questions for clarification. Keep an open mind.
4 Your own bias or prejudices; language differences or accents; noise and external distractions;

worry, fear, anger: not being able to focus; lack of attention span (due to tiredness, etc.)

5 Mental workload; distractions; the physical environment; physical demands; device/product design; process design
6 Understand why health-care staff make errors and, in particular, which 'systems factors' threaten patient safety; improve the safety culture of teams and organisations; enhance teamwork and improve communication between health-care staff; improve the design of healthcare systems and equipment; identify 'what went wrong' and predict 'what could go wrong'; appreciate how certain tools may help to lessen the likelihood of patient harm.

CHAPTER 9

Chapter 9 Test Your Knowledge

1 Assessment, evaluation, implementation, planning, diagnosis
2 Maintaining a safe environment, communication, breathing, eating and drinking, elimination, washing and dressing, controlling temperature, mobilisation, working and playing, expressing sexuality, sleeping, death and dying
3 Infection control, venous thrombolic embolism, falls, pressure ulcer (skin bundles), malnutrition screening tool
4 Next of kin
5 Glasgow Coma Scale (or Score)
6 Do not attempt resuscitation

CHAPTER 10

Activity 10.1

Respiratory rate:	
35 breaths per minute	scores 2
Oxygen saturation (SpO_2):	
89% on air	scores 2
Blood pressure:	
135/70 mmHg	scores 0
Heart rate:	
120 beats per minute	scores 1
Neuro response: Verbal	scores 1
Temperature: 38.2°C	scores 1
EWS: 7	

Activity 10.2

Situation: Hello Doctor. My name is Andros Pedro and I am the nurse in charge of J ward, looking after Mrs Jones, aged 82, who was admitted this morning with a chest infection. I am very concerned that Mrs Jones has now triggered an EWS score of 7.

Background: Mrs Jones has had one dose of her prescribed IV antibiotics and her EWS was recorded as 2 on admission. No oxygen therapy prescribed, as her oxygen saturations were assessed as being 93% on air.

Assessment: Mrs Jones' observations are:

Respiratory rate: 35 breaths per minute scores 2
Oxygen saturation (SpO_2): 89% on air scores 2
Blood pressure: 135/70 mmHg scores 0
Heart rate: 120 beats per minute scores 1
Neuro response: Verbal scores 1
Temperature: 38.2°C scores 1
EWS: 7

We are now presently administering 15 litres of oxygen therapy via a non-rebreathe mask and will perform observations half-hourly.

Recommendations: I would like you to review Mrs Jones urgently. What would you like me to do meanwhile? (i.e. blood gases, ECG recordings, etc.)

Activity 10.3

Stuporous: Suspension or great diminution of sensibility, as in disease or as caused by narcotics, intoxicants, etc.

Lethargic: Pertaining to, or affected with, lethargy; drowsy, sluggish.

Comatose: Relating to, or affected, with coma; unconscious.

Chapter 10 Test Your Knowledge

Situation: Hello Dr Jones, This is Jayne, a staff nurse on E ward. I'm concerned about Joe Smith who is having chest pain and his EWS is 4.

Background: He is 72, suffers with angina and was admitted to the ward 2 days ago following an episode of chest pain at home. This is the first episode of pain since admission; it started approximately 30 minutes ago and has not been relieved by GTN.

Assessment: His observations are RR 28 and SpO2 92% on air which is within the target prescribed. I am monitoring this continuously and will administer oxygen to keep within target. His HR is 114, BP 100 systolic. He is alert, blood glucose is 4.2, temperature 37 and he's pale and clammy.

Recommendation: Please can you come and see him now; we have done an ECG and cannulated him. Is there anything else you want us to do before you arrive?

CHAPTER 11

Chapter 11 Test Your Knowledge

1. See the list given in the chapter under the heading Nursing and Midwifery Council.
2. Root cause analysis
3. Civil courts
4. Criminal courts

5 The NMC to demonstrate fitness to practice and adherence to the code of conduct; your employer or trust to demonstrate fulfilment of your contractual agreement and that you are performing at the right standard for your role; the courts if there are claims of negligence or criminal acts; the patient and family.
6 Venous thrombolic embolism

CHAPTER 12

Activity 12.1

A concern is dealt with informally. The NHS trust you work for will have an Advice and Complaints Team (ACT) that will advise and assist the patient on achieving this type of outcome with appropriate staff.

A complaint formalises the issue. The Advice and Complaints Team will approach the areas concerned to gain a response within agreed timescales. The response will be sent from the Chief Executive.

Activity 12.2

1 Keep your distance
   - Maintain your personal space. Do not feel you have to stay in the same place and stand your ground.
   - Do look at the person, but do not stare/glare.
   - Avoid touching the other person.

2 Stay calm
   - If you are calm, you are in control. Stop for a moment before you speak. Control your breathing with deep breaths.
   - Don't take insults personally. You are the focus of the angry person's aggression, not the cause of it.

3 Let them speak
   - Is it possible to take them somewhere quiet? But do not put yourself at risk. Follow the agreed safety guidelines of your trust.
   - Give them the opportunity to talk.
   - Ask open questions: 'Tell me about it', 'What happened?'
   - Suspend judgement and remain neutral.

4 Let them know you are listening
   - Do not divide your attention between the person and another task.
   - Repeat what they have said to show you have understood.

5 Understand their position
   - Don't try to get yourself understood first.

6 Speak positively
   - Don't be tempted to score points, no matter how sorely tempted.
   - Don't use sarcasm.

7 Ask them to lower their voice
   - Remember, you do not have to accept offensive language or threats.

8 It isn't a sign of weakness to say sorry
   - You are not apologising for what you have done, you are empathising with the person.

9 Can a solution be found?
- No? Then explain why, sympathetically and clearly. Avoid jargon. Repeat the explanation if you have to. An angry person will probably not hear your first response.
- Is there an alternative solution you can offer?
- Do not make promises you cannot keep.

Chapter 12 Test Your Knowledge

1 A concern is dealt with informally. Your trust's will have an Advice and Complaints Team to advise and assist the patient. A complaint formalises the issue. The Advice and Complaints Team will approach the areas concerned, and the response will be sent from the Chief Executive.
2 Advice and Complaints Team
3 Communication with complainant unhelpful, ineffective, disrespectful
4 The National Patient Safety Agency (NPSA)
5 The Friends and Family Test
6 In your nursing portfolio

CHAPTER 13

Scenario One

1 During nurse handover; in a multi-disciplinary team meeting; in a quiet area away from the hustle and bustle of a busy ward. Ensure confidentiality; speak to the nurse in charge.
2 Use props to make conversation easier (photos, maps); draw or write things down on paper; stay calm; create a communication book that includes words, pictures and symbols; training around rehabilitation or work with a speech and language therapist (SALT).
3 Revise or devise a care plan with the patient using a person-centred approach; set realistic targets; revise and update plan on a regular basis.

Scenario Two

1 Greet the patient with a smile as you would normally do with anybody, and politely ask them for their name in order to book them in. You can engage them in a conversation out of interest and ask them to sit down. Make sure that the patient's personal details are correct and have been documented.

Scenario Three

1 Speak slowly and clearly; do not pretend to understand everything you hear: ask them to repeat and confirm information when necessary; don't be afraid to remind the person to slow down; think about the noise level/ distractions such as a radio or television, or transfer the call to another phone in a quieter area; learn telephone etiquette (manners); ask another member of staff.

Scenario Four: Staff Nurse

1. The patient.
2. To warn the patients that the clinic is running late.
3. Inform the patients. Give them the choice of waiting or making a new appointment. Rebook appointments for patients who are unable to stay.
4. Write on the information board that there is going to be a delay until 3.30 p.m. Apologise for the delay. Inform the patients as you are getting new information.

Scenario Four: Patient

1. Disorganised; people were arriving but there was no doctor. It shows poor communication and and there was a lack of information.
2. We should have been informed that there had been miscommunication initially and that the doctor would be available from 3.30 p.m. They should have apologised for the delay.
3. Yes, because people would have been arriving at different times thinking that they would be seen shortly. When people realised that no patients were being called there would have been angry situations. A notice could have been added to the information board informing patients of the delay.
4. We could have been shown where the vending machine is. Some patients may have diabetes. We could have been directed to the nearest toilet when necessary. We should have been offered the opportunity to make another appointment; for example, some people may have had to pick children up from school.
5. Good communication skills are required. If an extra clinic is being added in future, they should ensure that the doctor is informed and has it in their diary. The doctor could be reminded about the clinic 24 hours beforehand.

Scenario Five

1. Mohammed needs to be informed about his wife's operation and aftercare as he appears to have very limited knowledge. If Mohammed has been informed recently about his wife, has he actually understood what he was told? He may not understand all the medical terminology. His wife is also anxious, which will have an impact on her husband. He wants to know that she is having a halal diet.
2. She could undertake or review her customer awareness training.

Scenario Six

1. Karen needs to be informed that these patients are not children and should be treated with dignity and respect, calling them by their name, or title if preferred, rather than 'sweetheart'. She could attend a dementia workshop to update her skills or spend time working with a specialist nurse.

Scenario Seven

1 Report to the nurse in charge what you have observed on social media and block any further communication with that person.

Scenario Eight

1 Wait until there is a natural break in the tutorial and have a quiet word with the person to let them know that this is not acceptable behaviour. Inform the tutor that you are being distracted by another person using their mobile phone during the training session.

CHAPTER 14

Activity 14.1

1 Communication
2 Toileting
3 Pain relief
4 Nutrition and hydration

Chapter 14 Test Your Knowledge

1 Care, compassion, competence, communication, courage, commitment
2 Recommendation 276 One elderly but very lively patient who was a retired nurse herself told me:

> [A member of the nursing staff] who was in training doing the university course, I think, and she was doing a little spell on the ward, and on my first day she came and sat and chatted with me and talked about my experiences and my problem, and I enjoyed that, but that was the only time while I was in there that anybody came and talked to me.

Index

Communication Skills for Nurses, First Edition. Claire Boyd and Janet Dare

© 2014 John Wiley & Sons, Ltd. Published 2014 by John Wiley & Sons Ltd.

DEVELOPED BY STUDENTS FOR STUDENTS

You've made the right choice in selecting this Student Survival Skills book. Be sure to pick up the other books in the series to help you boost your competence both in the clinical skills lab and on your clinical placements – two core areas of your nursing education. The series is edited by Claire Boyd, a Practice Development Trainer in the Learning and Research Centre at North Bristol Healthcare Trust in the UK working closely with a team of practicing nurses and nursing students. Therefore, each handy pocket-sized book in the series includes words of wisdom and advice for real-life situations.

The Student Survival Skills books are:

- Developed by students, for students
- Clear, straightforward, and jargon-free
- Tied in with the NMC standards for pre-registration education and the Essential Skills Clusters
- Filled with examples and questions based on real life nursing and healthcare situations
- Available in a range of digital formats

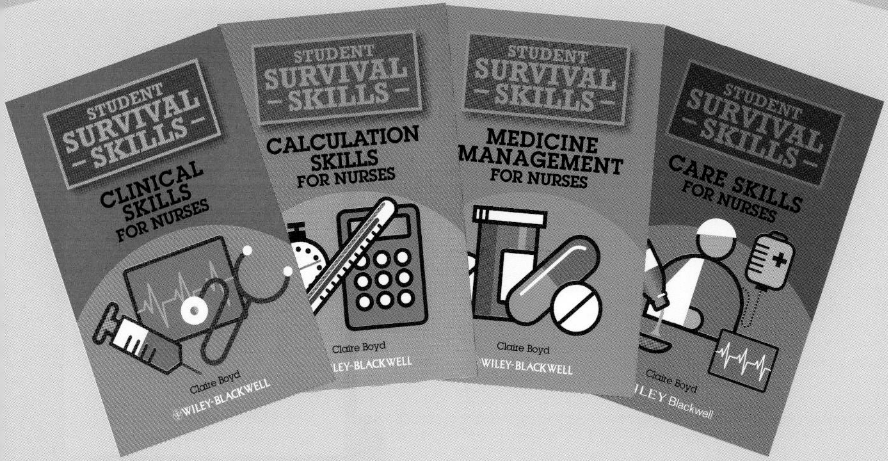

Clinical Skills for Nurses
2013 • 224 pages
9781118448779

Calculation Skills for Nurses
2013 • 208 pages
9781118448892

Medicine Management Skills for Nurses
2013 • 280 pages
9781118448854

Care Skills for Nurses
2013 • 216 pages
9781118657386

Communication Skills for Nurses
2014 • 256 pages
9781118767528

Study Skills for Nurses
2014 • 240 pages
9781118657430

13-58843

Digital editions are available for download to your computer or e-book reader. Please visit **www.wiley.com** or your preferred e-book vendor for further details or to purchase.

WILEY

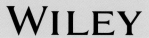

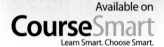

Available on
CourseSmart
Learn Smart. Choose Smart.

Wiley E-Text
Powered by VitalSource®

More and more titles from Wiley Nursing are now available in interactive ebook formats, such as **Wiley E-Text**, featuring downloadable text and images, highlighting and note-taking facilities, book-marking, cross-referencing, in-text searching, and linking to references and glossary terms.

Many titles are now also available instantly on **CourseSmart**. CourseSmart offers a range of study tools and the flexibility of digital textbook rental.

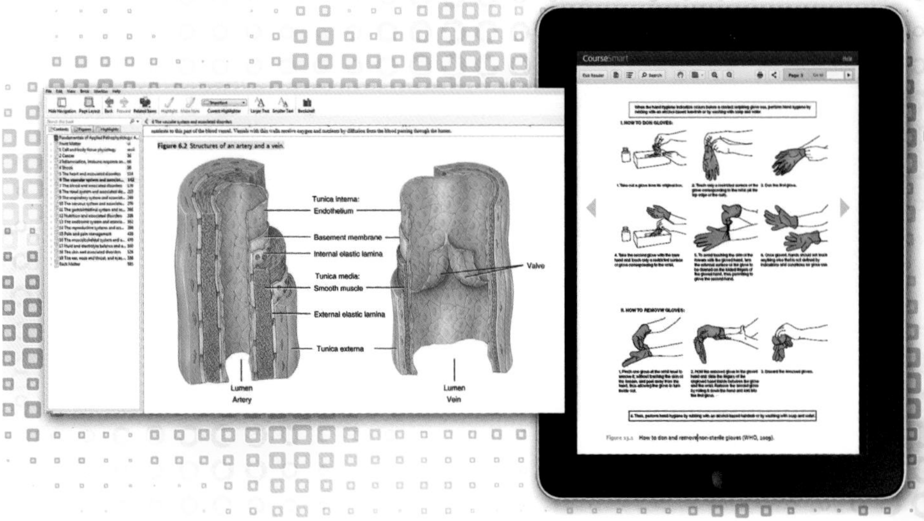

For more details, and to discover these titles, visit:

www.wileynursing.com and
www.coursesmart.com

WILEY